Preparing for Terrorism

Tools for Evaluating the Metropolitan Medical Response System Program

Frederick J. Manning and Lewis Goldfrank, *Editors*

Committee on Evaluation of the Metropolitan Medical Response System Program

Board on Health Sciences Policy

INSTITUTE OF MEDICINE

NATIONAL ACADEMY PRESS
Washington, D.C.

NATIONAL ACADEMY PRESS • 2101 Constitution Avenue, NW • Washington, DC 20418

NOTICE: The project that is the subject of this report was approved by the Governing Board of the National Research Council, whose members are drawn from the councils of the National Academy of Sciences, the National Academy of Engineering, and the Institute of Medicine. The members of the committee responsible for this report were chosen for their special competences and with regard for appropriate balance.

Support for this project was provided by the Office of Emergency Preparedness, U.S. Department of Health and Human Services (Contract No. 282-99-0045, TO#5). This support does not constitute endorsement of the views expressed in the report.

Library of Congress Cataloging-in-Publication Data

Institute of Medicine (U.S.). Committee on Evaluation of the Metropolitan Medical Response Program.
Preparing for terrorism : tools for evaluating the Metropolitan Medical Response System program / Frederick J. Manning and Lewis Goldfrank, editors ; Committee on Evaluation of the Metropolitan Medical Response System Program, Board on Health Sciences Policy, Institute of Medicine.
p. ; cm.
Includes bibliographical references.
ISBN 0-309-08428-8 (pbk.)
1. Disaster medicine. 2. Emergency medical services. 3. Terrorism—Health aspects. 4. Weapons of mass destruction—Health aspects. 5. Emergency management. 6. Health planning.
[DNLM: 1. Disaster Planning—organization & administration. 2. Emergency Medical Services—organization & administration. 3. Health Planning. 4. Program Evaluation—methods. 5. Terrorism. WX 185 I59p 2002] I. Manning, Frederick J. II. Goldfrank, Lewis R., 1941- III. Title.
RA645.5 .I54 2002
362.18—dc21

2002007502

Additional copies of this report are available for sale from the National Academy Press, 2101 Constitution Avenue, NW, Box 285, Washington, DC 20055. Call (800) 624-6242 or (202) 334-3313 (in the Washington metropolitan area), or visit the NAP's on-line bookstore at **www.nap.edu.**

The full text of the report is available on-line at **www.nap.edu**

For more information about the Institute of Medicine, visit the IOM home page at **www.iom.edu.**

Printed in the United States of America.

The serpent has been a symbol of long life, healing, and knowledge among almost all cultures and religions since the beginning of recorded history. The serpent adopted as a logotype by the Institute of Medicine is a relief carving from ancient Greece, now held by the Staatliche Museen in Berlin.

First Printing, July 2002
Second Printing, May 2003

"Knowing is not enough; we must apply.
Willing is not enough; we must do."
—Goethe

INSTITUTE OF MEDICINE

Shaping the Future for Health

THE NATIONAL ACADEMIES

National Academy of Sciences
National Academy of Engineering
Institute of Medicine
National Research Council

The **National Academy of Sciences** is a private, nonprofit, self-perpetuating society of distinguished scholars engaged in scientific and engineering research, dedicated to the furtherance of science and technology and to their use for the general welfare. Upon the authority of the charter granted to it by the Congress in 1863, the Academy has a mandate that requires it to advise the federal government on scientific and technical matters. Dr. Bruce M. Alberts is president of the National Academy of Sciences.

The **National Academy of Engineering** was established in 1964, under the charter of the National Academy of Sciences, as a parallel organization of outstanding engineers. It is autonomous in its administration and in the selection of its members, sharing with the National Academy of Sciences the responsibility for advising the federal government. The National Academy of Engineering also sponsors engineering programs aimed at meeting national needs, encourages education and research, and recognizes the superior achievements of engineers. Dr. Wm. A. Wulf is president of the National Academy of Engineering.

The **Institute of Medicine** was established in 1970 by the National Academy of Sciences to secure the services of eminent members of appropriate professions in the examination of policy matters pertaining to the health of the public. The Institute acts under the responsibility given to the National Academy of Sciences by its congressional charter to be an adviser to the federal government and, upon its own initiative, to identify issues of medical care, research, and education. Dr. Kenneth I. Shine is president of the Institute of Medicine.

The **National Research Council** was organized by the National Academy of Sciences in 1916 to associate the broad community of science and technology with the Academy's purposes of furthering knowledge and advising the federal government. Functioning in accordance with general policies determined by the Academy, the Council has become the principal operating agency of both the National Academy of Sciences and the National Academy of Engineering in providing services to the government, the public, and the scientific and engineering communities. The Council is administered jointly by both Academies and the Institute of Medicine. Dr. Bruce M. Alberts and Dr. Wm. A. Wulf are chairman and vice chairman, respectively, of the National Research Council.

COMMITTEE ON EVALUATION OF THE METROPOLITAN MEDICAL RESPONSE SYSTEM PROGRAM

LEWIS GOLDFRANK (*Chair*), Director, Emergency Medicine, New York University Medical Center, Bellevue Hospital Center, New York, New York

JOSEPH BARBERA, Director, Disaster Medicine Program, The George Washington University, Washington, DC

GEORGES C. BENJAMIN, Secretary, Maryland Department of Health and Mental Hygiene, Baltimore, Maryland

JAMES BENTLEY, Senior Vice President, Strategic Policy Planning, American Hospital Association, Washington, DC

KENNETH I. BERNS, President and CEO, Mount Sinai Medical Center, New York, New York

RAYMOND M. DOWNEY, Battalion Chief and Chief of Rescue Operations, Special Operations Command, Fire Department, City of New York (from November 2000 to September 2001)

FRANCES EDWARDS-WINSLOW, Director, Office of Emergency Services, San Jose, California

LINDA F. FAIN, Disaster Mental Health Consultant, Auburn, California

FRED HENRETIG, Director, Clinical Toxicology, and Director, Poison Control Center, Children's Hospital of Philadelphia, Pennsylvania

DARRELL HIGUCHI, Deputy Chief, Los Angeles County Fire Department, Los Angeles, California (from November 2001)

ARNOLD HOWITT, Executive Director, Taubman Center, Kennedy School of Government, Harvard University, Cambridge, Massachusetts

LAURA LEVITON, Senior Program Officer for Research and Evaluation, Robert Wood Johnson Foundation, Princeton, New Jersey

WILLIAM MYERS, Health Commissioner, Columbus, Ohio

DENNIS M. PERROTTA, State Epidemiologist and Chief, Bureau of Epidemiology, Texas Department of Health, Austin, Texas

JEFFREY L. RUBIN, Chief, Disaster Medical Services Division, Emergency Medical Services Authority, State of California, Sacramento, California

AMY E. SMITHSON, Senior Associate, Henry L. Stimson Center, Washington, DC (from November 2000 to July 2001)

DARREL STEPHENS, Chief, Charlotte-Mecklenburg Police Department, Charlotte, North Carolina

Board on Health Sciences Policy Liaison

BERNARD GOLDSTEIN, Dean, Graduate School of Public Health, University of Pittsburgh, Pittsburgh, Pennsylvania

Study Staff

FREDERICK J. MANNING, Study Director
REBECCA LOEFFLER, Project Assistant

Institute of Medicine Staff

ANDREW POPE, Director, Board on Health Sciences Policy
ALDEN CHANG II, Administrative Assistant, Board on Health Sciences Policy
CARLOS GABRIEL, Financial Associate

Consultant

LAUREN SCHIFF, Incident Commander and Operations Officer, Appalachian Search and Rescue Conference, Charlottesville, Virginia.

Independent Report Reviewers

This report has been reviewed in draft form by individuals chosen for their diverse perspectives and technical expertise, in accordance with procedures approved by the National Research Council's Report Review Committee. The purpose of this independent review is to provide candid and critical comments that will assist the institution in making its published report as sound as possible and to ensure that the report meets institutional standards for objectivity, evidence, and responsiveness to the study charge. The contents of the review comments and draft manuscript remain confidential to protect the integrity of the deliberative process. We wish to thank the following individuals for their participation in the review of this report:

MARTIN BLASER, Professor of Internal Medicine and Chair, Department of Medicine, New York University
GREGORY M. BOGDAN, Research Director and Medical Toxicology Coordinator, Rocky Mountain Poison Center, Denver, Colorado
BARRY S. COLLER, David Rockefeller Professor of Medicine, Physician-in-Chief, The Rockefeller University Hospital, and Vice President for Medical Affairs, The Rockefeller University, New York, New York
GEORGE R. FLORES, Director of Public Health, San Diego Department of Health, San Diego, California
VINCENT T. FRANCISCO, Associate Director, Work Group on Health Promotion and Community Development, University of Kansas, Lawrence, Kansas

ROBERT MALSON, President, District of Columbia Hospital Association, Washington, D.C.

PAUL M. MANISCALCO, Past President, National Association of Emergency Medical Technicians

PETER ROSEN, Director, Emergency Medicine Residency Program, Department of Emergency Medicine, University of California, San Diego School of Medicine

ROBERT E. SHOPE, Professor of Pathology, University of Texas Medical Branch, Galveston, Texas

Although the reviewers listed above have provided many constructive comments and suggestions, they were not asked to endorse the conclusions or recommendations nor did they see the final draft of the report before its release. The review of this report was overseen by **LESTER N. WRIGHT,** Chief Medical Officer, New York Department of Correctional Services, Albany, New York, appointed by the Institute of Medicine, and **ALEXANDER H. FLAX,** Consultant, Potomac, Maryland, appointed by the NRC's Report Review Committee. These individuals were responsible for making certain that an independent examination of this report was carried out in accordance with institutional procedures and that all review comments were carefully considered. Responsibility for the final content of this report rests entirely with the authoring committee and the institution.

This report is dedicated to Ray Downey, Chief of Rescue Operations, Fire Department, City of New York, our friend and colleague on this Institute of Medicine committee, killed in the line of duty while leading rescue efforts at the World Trade Center after the terrorist attack on September 11, 2001.

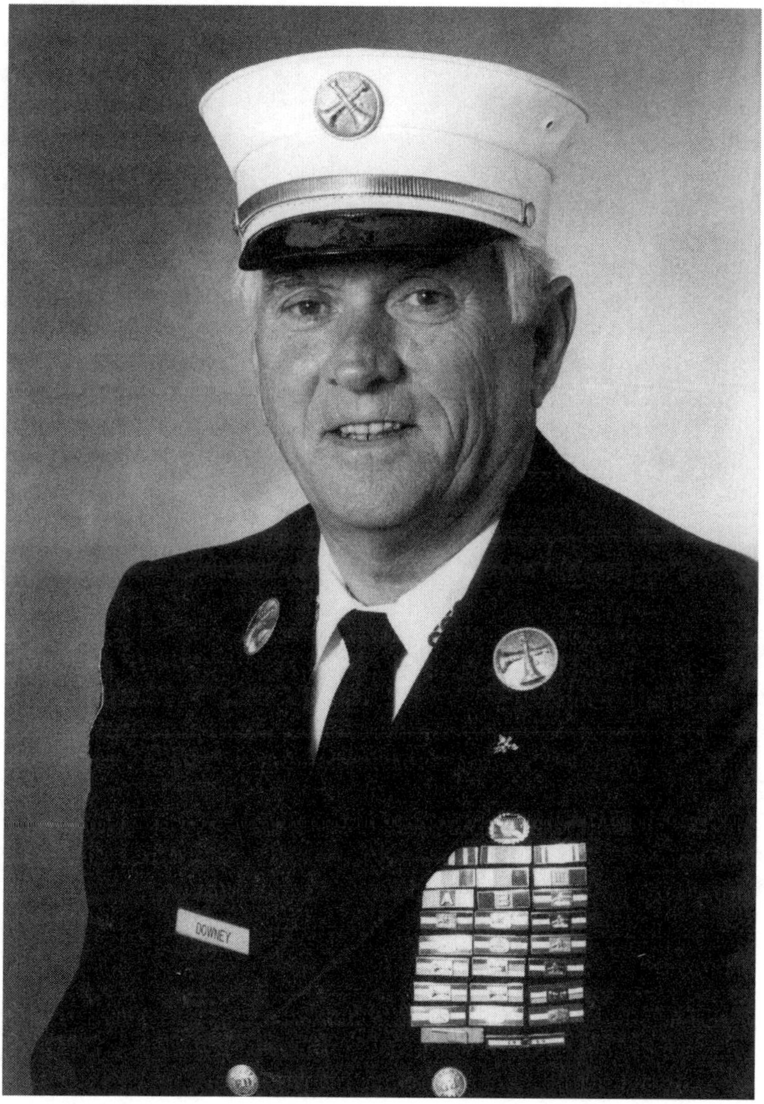

Preface

Having a vision, a mission, and a passion are invariably seen as conditions for success. The 1995 U.S. Department of Health and Human Services (DHHS) concept of a Metropolitan Medical Response System (MMRS) demonstrated that the leaders of DHHS had a vision for an effective response to a mass-casualty terrorism incident with a weapon of mass destruction. The mission was to expand the experimental model of the Metropolitan Medical Strike Team (MMST) established in Washington, D.C., and neighboring counties into a national program.

The problem that the Office of Emergency Preparedness (OEP) of DHHS faced was the dilemma of knowing what preparedness is and determining whether preparedness could be recognized if it was achieved. Under these circumstances, OEP requested that the Institute of Medicine determine how effective this MMRS program effort is and how valuable it could become.

A typically diverse Institute of Medicine working group consisting of leaders, strategists, practitioners, and analysts of societal needs in terms of readiness for disasters and terrorism with weapons of mass destruction was established in the autumn of 2000. Over the following 18 months we constructed a diversified analytic program that emphasizes continuous quality improvement to enhance relationships, understanding, and services, and improve equipment and personnel in the pursuit of preparedness. Our approach is based on the belief that all services are valuable, that they must be integrated, and that shared leadership with democratic, open management approaches will effectively be able to use each metropolitan region's assets. We have suggested that document and data analysis, site visits by a team of expert peer reviewers, and observations of exercises and drills be used to analyze a region's accomplishments.

Some committee members' theoretical approaches to the requirements of this project as well as the limited cooperative spirit seen in some MMRS program efforts were initial concerns for the committee. These limitations to the committee's potential were dramatically altered by the September 2001 assault that toppled the World Trade Center and paralyzed the U.S. aviation system and by the mailing of anthrax-laden letters in October 2001 that almost toppled the U.S. public health and postal systems. The events led to the tragic death of a fellow committee member, Ray Downey, Chief of Rescue Operations, Fire Department, City of New York, and thousands of other Americans. These terrorist acts led to a disruption of the equanimity not just of New York City but of our entire country. Our committee, recognizing the timeliness and exceptional importance of our task, responded with the necessary passion to complete the tasks of this analytic process.

We believe that this product will allow OEP, state and federal governments, and all who create preparedness teams to offer a more informed, qualified, and integrated approach to preparedness and public health. This report will be an essential tool in analyses of the depth and breadth of governmental performance and interagency collaboration. This effort—and in particular, U.S. society's recognition of the importance of our goals—will allow us to save lives and property in future biological, chemical, and radiological terrorist events. The vision was of vital importance. We hope that our passion has allowed us to accomplish the mission and that OEP will have the tools that it needs to determine if we in America are ready to protect ourselves from unknown potential assaults and will remain so for the future.

Lewis R. Goldfrank
Chair

Acronyms and Abbreviations

ARC	American Red Cross
CAR	Capability Assessment for Readiness
CBR	chemical, biological, and radiological
CBRDT	Chemical/Biological Rapid Deployment Team
CDC	Centers for Disease Control and Prevention
CDP	Center for Domestic Preparedness (U.S. Department of Justice)
CHER-CAP	Comprehensive HAZMAT Emergency Response-Capability Assessment Program
CSEPP	Chemical Stockpile Emergency Preparedness Program
DHHS	U.S. Department of Health and Human Services
DMAT	Disaster Medical Assistance Team
DMORT	Disaster Mortuary Team
DOD	U.S. Department of Defense
DOE	U.S. Department of Energy
DOJ	U.S. Department of Justice
DVA	U.S. Department of Veterans Affairs
ED	emergency department
EOC	Emergency Operations Center
EOP	emergency operations plan
EMAC	emergency management assistance compact
EMI	Emergency Management Institute

EMS	emergency medical services
EPA	Environmental Protection Agency
ESF	emergency support functions
FBI	Federal Bureau of Investigation
FEMA	Federal Emergency Management Agency
FRP	Federal Response Plan
FY	fiscal year
GAO	General Accounting Office
Hazmat	hazardous materials
HDS	Hazardous Devices School
HMO	health maintenance organization
IOM	Institute of Medicine
JCAHCO	Joint Commission for Accreditation of Healthcare Organizations
LCAR	Local Capability Assessment for Readiness
LEPC	Local Emergency Planning Committee
MEMA	Maryland Emergency Management Agency
MMRS	Metropolitan Medical Response System
MMST	Metropolitan Medical Strike Team
MOU	memorandum of understanding
NAPA	National Academy of Public Administration
NCP	National Contingency Plan or National Oil and Hazardous Substances Contingency Plan
NDMS	National Disaster Medical System
NDPC	National Domestic Preparedness Consortium
NDPO	National Domestic Preparedness Office
NEMA	National Emergency Management Association
NMRT	National Medical Response Team
OCFD	Oklahoma City Fire Department
OCPD	Oklahoma City Police Department
ODP	Office of Domestic Preparedness (U.S. Department of Justice)
OEP	Office of Emergency Preparedness
OES	Office of Emergency Services

OMB	Office of Management and Budget
OSHA	Occupational Safety and Health Administration
OSLDPS	Office of State and Local Domestic Preparedness Support
POC	point of contact
REP	Radiological Emergency Preparedness Program (Federal Emergency Management Agency)
ROC	Regional Operations Center
SOP	standard operating procedure
USAR	U.S. Army Reserve
USNRC	U.S. Nuclear Regulatory Commission
VA	Department of Veterans Affairs
VMI	vendor-managed inventory
WMD	weapons of mass destruction

Contents

LIST OF TABLES, FIGURES, AND BOX

Tables

Figures

Box

Preparing for Terrorism

Executive Summary

Abstract: *The Metropolitan Medical Response System (MMRS) program of the U.S. Department of Health and Human Services (DHHS) provides funds to major U.S. cities to help them develop plans for coping with the health and medical consequences of a terrorist attack with chemical, biological, or radiological (CBR) agents.*

The DHHS Office of Emergency Preparedness (OEP) asked the Institute of Medicine (IOM) to assist in assessing the effectiveness of the MMRS program by identifying or developing performance measures and systems and then using those measures to establish appropriate evaluation methods, tools, and processes for use by OEP to assess both its own management of the program and local preparedness in the cities that have participated in the program.

Both the MMRS program and the local preparedness to cope with terrorism that it seeks to enhance can and should be improved by a comprehensive evaluation program. Since the nature of the threat of CBR attack and U.S. cities both undergo continual change, preparedness to respond to a CBR attack must also undergo continual change. Therefore, it is important to conceptualize preparedness as a continual process rather than the achievement of a single final plan. The evaluation of preparedness must necessarily, therefore, also be a continual process rather than a one-time event or even a series of events spaced at long time intervals.

This report provides a set of measurement tools and describes a process for evaluating the extent to which communities have implemented the plans required by the MMRS program and have begun to achieve real preparedness. Specifically, the committee lists 23 essential capabilities that form the basis for preparedness. For each of those capabilities, the committee provides a small set of pre-

paredness indicators by which community preparedness can be judged and advice on a suitable method for gathering the necessary data with which a proper conclusion can be drawn.

In summary, this report provides the managers of the MMRS program and others concerned about local capabilities to cope with CBR terrorism with three evaluation tools and a three-part assessment method. The tools provided are a questionnaire survey eliciting feedback about the management of the MMRS program, a table of preparedness indicators for 23 essential response capabilities, and a set of three scenarios and related questions for group discussion. The assessment method described integrates document inspection, a site visit by a team of expert peer reviewers, and observations at community exercises and drills.

Among the many federal efforts to combat terrorism is the Metropolitan Medical Response System (MMRS) program of the U.S. Department of Health and Human Services (DHHS), which attempts to enhance the preparedness of major U.S. cities with regard to the health and medical consequences of an attack or threatened attack with chemical, biological, or radiological (CBR) agents.

The DHHS Office of Emergency Preparedness (OEP) has been contracting with the most heavily populated U.S. cities since 1997 in an effort to improve those cities' capabilities to respond to terrorism incidents on the scale of the September 11, 2001, attacks on the World Trade Center and the Pentagon. The central focus of this effort, the MMRS program, has been on unfamiliar chemical and biological agents, although many of the requisite capabilities for dealing with the consequences of those agents are necessary for an effective response to an attack with explosives or radiological agents as well or even for an effective response to natural disasters. The contracts, which OEP has signed with 122 cities as of the spring of 2002, provide funds for special equipment and a cache of pharmaceuticals and medical supplies, and in turn demand detailed plans on how the city will organize and respond to chemical and biological terrorism incidents. A large number of these cities have now produced acceptable plans, and OEP turned to IOM for assistance in evaluating the extent to which its efforts and these plans have actually prepared cities to cope with the consequences of mass-casualty terrorism with a CBR agent (i.e., are the cities now well-prepared, and how has OEP contributed?).

CHARGE TO THE COMMITTEE

OEP asked the Institute of Medicine (IOM) to assist OEP in assessing the effectiveness of the MMRS program by identifying or developing performance measures and systems and identifying barriers related to the MMRS development process. IOM was then to use those measures to establish appropriate evaluation methods, tools, and processes for use by OEP. In response to that request, IOM formed the Committee on Evaluation of the Metropolitan Medical Response System Program.

The primary measure of effectiveness for any program is the extent to which it achieves its ultimate goals. Therefore, in Phase I of this project the Committee identified almost 500 preparedness indicators that might be used to assess the response capabilities of MMRS program cities at the site, jurisdictional, and governmental levels. Those indicators are described in the committee's Phase I report (Institute of Medicine, 2001) and are reprinted as Appendix E of this report. In Phase II, the committee used the preparedness indicators established in Phase I to develop usable evaluation methods, tools, and processes for assessing both program management by OEP and the capabilities of the local communities necessary for effective response to CBR terrorism. Those methods, tools, and processes are the subject of this report.

CHEMICAL, BIOLOGICAL, AND RADIOLOGICAL WEAPONS

There are thousands of chemicals that may result in morbidity or mortality for humans at some dose. In the present context, "chemical agents" are generally considered to be a relatively short list of chemicals that have at some time been "weaponized" for military use. Some of these agents have no other use (e.g., nerve agents and mustard gas); other agents such as chlorine and ammonia are in wide use in industry. Often classified by the site or nature of their effects in humans as nerve, blister, choking, vomiting, and tear agents and incapacitants, many of these chemicals are poorly understood by civilian hazardous materials technicians and other emergency responders, medical personnel, and law enforcement officials. The agents listed below have been the primary focus of efforts to prepare for chemical terrorism, in part because of their toxicities but to a greater extent because of the health care community's unfamiliarity with these agents:

- Nerve agents
  - Tabun (GA)
  - Sarin (GB)
  - Soman (GD)
  - GF
  - VX
- Vesicants (blister agents)
  - Mustard (H, HD)
  - Lewisite (L)
  - Phosgene oxime (CX)

- Blood agents
    - Hydrocyanic acid (AC)
    - Cyanogen chloride (CK)
    - Arsine
    - Methyl isocyanate
- Choking agents
    - Phosgene (CG, DP)
    - Chlorine
    - Ammonia

Biological agents with adverse effects on human health include viruses, bacteria, fungi, and toxins. The distinguishing feature of biological agents other than toxins is their ability to propagate—exposure to an extremely small amount can lead to an overwhelming infection, and in some cases the victim may even become a source of infection for additional victims. This propagation within the exposed person (that is, incubation) takes time, however, so the effects of viruses, bacteria, and fungi may not become apparent until days or weeks after the initial exposure. There may be no obvious temporal or geographical concentration of victims to help medical personnel arrive at a diagnosis and make law enforcement personnel suspect a crime. Diagnosis of infection in individual patients will also be rendered more difficult because most of the agents considered to be likely threats are very rarely seen in U.S. cities and the initial symptoms that they produce (fever, headache, general malaise) are also characteristic of those produced by many common diseases. As difficult as it was to contain the spread of anthrax from just a few spore-filled letters in the autumn of 2001, the fact that the letters announced the presence of anthrax spores actually made the diagnosis and response far easier than if, for example, the perpetrator had covertly introduced spores into the air-handling system of a sports arena or airport. The victims in that case would have dispersed, perhaps very widely, by the time they became ill, and many might have died before an accurate diagnosis could have been made.

As in the case of chemicals, would-be terrorists have a large number of potentially harmful biological agents from which to choose. Indeed, the tools of biotechnology might even be used to make some biological variants that have not previously existed, so to suggest that would-be terrorists will only use agents that have been the focus of military weapons programs would be folly. The agents that have been developed as biological weapons were carefully selected for their suitability as weapons, however, and few civilian American physicians have experience in either the diagnosis or treatment of the diseases caused by those agents. For that reason, these agents have been the focus of counterterrorism training and other preparations. The specific agents that MMRS cities are directed to consider in their planning are those responsible for anthrax, botulism, hemorrhagic fever, plague, smallpox, and tularemia.

The term "radiological weapon," in distinction to nuclear weapon, refers to a weapon that would disseminate radioactive materials by means other than an uncontrolled fission chain reaction. The so-called dirty bomb, which consists of radioactive material wrapped around conventional explosives, is the best-known example. Exposure to excessive amounts of radiation does not make one radioactive, but in the short run it can produce skin reddening and loss of hair, nausea and vomiting, diarrhea, sterility, tissue fibrosis, organ atrophy, bone marrow failure, and death. These effects are not instantaneous, so radiological terrorism would present some of the same challenges for clinical diagnosis and law enforcement as biological terrorism. Some of these effects may be transient, but the genes of some exposed individuals may also damaged, leading to cancer or birth defects in their offspring that are manifest only years later.

Decay of the commonly used radioactive materials is very slow, so contamination is a serious clinical concern. Although not invisible, a finely ground or powdered agent could be detected and removed only with the aid of special equipment for detection and decontamination. Activities required to cope with a radiological incident may resemble those required to cope with either a chemical incident or a biological incident, depending on whether the attack is overt (perhaps a conventional bomb wrapped in highly radioactive material) or covert (introduction of radioactive dust into an air, water, or food supply).

THE MMRS PROGRAM

Perhaps because the immediate stimulus for the MMRS program was an incident involving the release of a military nerve agent in the Tokyo subway in 1995, the first two Metropolitan Medical "Strike Teams" were essentially enhanced hazardous materials (hazmat) teams; and their plans, training, and equipment focused on the demands of coping with potential events involving chemical agent. Some of the other early MMRS program cities changed the strike team concept by integrating strike team capabilities into existing fire department, emergency medical services, and police training and organizational infrastructures. In addition, their plans incorporated local public health officials; nongovernmental organizations; state agencies, including the National Guard; federal military and nonmilitary officials; and private health care organizations. OEP soon amended the initial contracts to focus more attention on coping with a covert release of a biological agent and changed the name of the program to the Metropolitan Medical Response System. The new name emphasizes that the program is intended to enhance the capabilities of existing systems that involve not just hazmat personnel, law enforcement personnel, emergency medical services personnel, public hospitals, and the American Red Cross but also public health agencies and laboratories, private hospitals, clinics, independent physicians, and other private-sector organizations. This emphasis on enhancing existing systems rather than creating new, and perhaps competing, CBR weapon-specific systems was strongly recommended by a previous IOM committee as a first principle in efforts to prepare for CBR terrorism (Institute of Medicine, 1999).

EXISTING EMERGENCY RESPONSE SYSTEMS

A previous IOM study (Institute of Medicine, 1999) pointed out that despite the justifiable emphasis on the novel aspects of a possible terrorist attack with a chemical or biological agent, frameworks for responding to incidents of both types already exist. It argued that strengthening existing mechanisms for dealing with unintentional releases of hazardous chemicals, for monitoring food safety, for detecting and responding to infectious disease outbreaks, and for coping with natural disasters with large numbers of casualties is preferable to building a new system focused solely on potentially devastating but low-probability terrorist events.

The all-hazards approach currently advocated by emergency managers requires the availability of systems capable of responding not only to high-probability hazards but also to unexpected events. Those systems include individuals and organizations, means for communication and collaboration among those entities, procedures for the monitoring of public health on a regular basis, and the availability of appropriate equipment to protect responders and save life and property. No universal standard currently exists to define the concept of an "adequate" capacity of municipal emergency management, and U.S. metropolitan areas have a wide range of capabilities

The core of emergency management is at the local or regional level and follows a bottom-up approach. Historically, local medical and public health personnel have been the first to notice and respond to rare or unique symptoms and slowly developing trends among victims. In addition, local leaders are the ones most likely to understand local priorities and the implications of critical decisions for their communities. In parallel to the fact that the core of emergency management is at the local level, one of the distinguishing features of the MMRS program is that it is not just a new or better way of providing federal aid to stricken communities but is also a way to help communities themselves deal both with the initial stages of a disaster and with the subsequent influx of outside assistance. Therefore, strengthening existing systems not only improves the emergency response to terrorist incidents but also improves the emergency responses to other disasters.

OTHER FEDERAL PROGRAMS TO STRENGTHEN LOCAL CAPABILITIES

The federal government is prepared to provide a substantial amount and diverse forms of assistance to communities stricken by a disaster. With a few exceptions, however, none of this assistance will be available to the affected community until at least 12 to 24 hours after it is requested (and the request itself may not come for hours or even days after the initiating event, be it an earthquake, a flood, or the release of a CBR agent). In contrast, as noted above, the MMRS program provides proactive, pre-disaster assistance; it is not a federal response. It provides funds for the purchase of special CBR agent-specific equipment, supplies, and pharmaceuticals for local law enforcement, fire department, and emergency medical personnel, while it demands substantial integrated planning by the local partners.

An important element of that planning and an important consideration in any attempt to measure the impact of the MMRS program is the fact that at least four other federal entities provide additional equipment and CBR agent-specific training: the U.S. Department of Justice Office of Domestic Preparedness (formerly the Office of State and Local Domestic Preparedness Support), the Federal Bureau of Investigation, the Centers for Disease Control and Prevention, and the Federal Emergency Management Agency. In past years, the U.S. Department of Defense was a major source of training and equipment for the largest U.S. cities. Chapter 3 describes these programs, in which nearly all MMRS program cities participated. A significant consequence of this multitude of programs of special importance to the work of the Committee is that it effectively precludes unequivocal assignment of credit for local preparedness.

FEEDBACK TO OEP ON PROGRAM MANAGEMENT

Part of the charge to the committee concerns the performance of OEP staff in their administration of the MMRS program. That is, how can OEP determine at the program (i.e., national) level whether the strategies, resources, mechanisms, technical assistance, and monitoring processes provided to the MMRS development process are effective? The question of effectiveness obviously cannot be fully answered independently of some measure of the capabilities of the MMRS program communities, but it is nevertheless possible to make some judgments about OEP's administration of the program by asking whether its contracts cover all the activities necessary for effective response. The committee in fact identified a number of shortfalls in this regard. Perhaps more valuable sources of feedback on this issue are OEP's contractors, that is, the MMRS program communities, which can provide information about the extent to which they used OEP technical assistance and resources in fulfilling the terms of their contracts, their perceptions of its value, and the extent to which fulfilling the terms of the contract actually improved community preparedness. To this end the committee provides an initial evaluation tool: a questionnaire survey for administration to OEP's primary point of contact in each MMRS program community.

The initial section of the proposed survey, which could be administered at any point in the course of the contract or after the completion of the contract, solicits input on the extent to which an MMRS program community used OEP-provided resources in fulfilling the terms of its contract and how useful it found those resources for that purpose. The survey then queries the respondent about the perceived abilities of the community in a number of functional areas that the committee believes are essential to preparedness. It concludes with several open-ended questions regarding remaining barriers to preparedness for a terrorist attack with a CBR weapon and changes in the day-to-day and disaster-oriented operations of the public safety, public health, and health services agencies in the community.

FEEDBACK TO OEP ON PROGRAM SUCCESS

Regardless of how the MMRS program is managed by OEP, the ultimate test of the program's worth lies in how well it has helped local communities prepare for the consequences of a massive terrorist attack with CBR weapons. The survey described above begins to answer that question by soliciting the opinions of the MMRS program communities themselves. Complementing that approach are the committee's recommendations for an independent and systematic assessment of the response capabilities of the large metropolitan areas that have participated in or that will participate in the MMRS program. Those recommendations call for a three-part process composed of periodic review of documents and records, on-site assessment by a team of peers, and observation of community-initiated exercises and drills. Together the three components provide the means for assessing 23 essential capabilities necessary for any community to respond effectively to the wide variety of CBR terrorism incidents that it may suffer.

Essential Capabilities

The committee believes that effective response to incidents involving CBR weapons of any sort will require every community to make plans and develop expertise in 23 distinct activities. No single activity is necessarily more important than the others, and the specific characteristics and importance of these 23 essential response capabilities vary with the type of agent, as do the relative importances of the various capabilities, but together they form a comprehensive picture of the preparedness of the community.

1. Relationship development (partnering)
2. Communication system development
3. Hazard assessment
4. Training
5. Equipment and supplies
6. Mass immunization and prophylaxis
7. Addressing the information needs of the public and the news media
8. First responder protection
9. Rescue and stabilization of victims
10. Diagnosis and agent identification
11. Decontamination of victims (at site of exposure or at hospital or treatment site)
12. Transportation of victims
13. Distribution of supplies, equipment, and pharmaceuticals
14. Shelter and feeding of evacuated and displaced persons
15. Definitive medical care
16. Mental health services for responders, victims, caregivers, and their families
17. Volunteer utilization and control
18. Crowd and traffic control
19. Evacuation and quarantine decisions and operations
20. Fatality management
21. Environmental cleanup, physical restoration of facilities, and certification of safety
22. Follow-up study of responder, caregiver, and victim health
23. Process for continuous evaluation of needs and resources

Because not all of these capabilities are addressed in the MMRS program contracts, and the Committee was seeking to measure not contract compliance but actual preparedness, the Committee chose to build its evaluation program on these 23 essential capabilities rather than the 12 "deliverables" demanded by the MMRS program contracts. Consistent with the committee's earlier endorsement of an all-hazards approach, all are relevant and necessary elements of responses to disasters of all kinds, natural and technological, deliberate and inadvertent. For each of these 23 capabilities, the committee derived one or more measures or preparedness indicators that could be sought in any community.

Preparedness Indicators

The products demanded of the communities with MMRS program contracts are for the most part written plans, and although written plans are certainly necessary elements of preparedness, they are in most cases only the beginning of a continuous process. Some elements of these plans can be implemented only during or after an actual incident or a very realistic exercise; but many require advance preparations, such as the purchase of equipment, hiring and training of personnel, or even changes in the way in which routine operations are conducted (for example, citywide electronic surveillance of emergency department visits or 911 calls). Even though these advance preparations and their documentation are necessary for preparedness, they are not the same sort of performances that might be assessed in an actual mass-casualty event (whether it involves CBR terrorism or not) or a drill or field exercise. Measures related to advance preparations are generally easier and cheaper to access, however, and can provide a measure of effective response capability or potential (although in the absence of regular acts of mass-casualty-producing CBR terrorism, no data can validate the relationship between the selected indicators and actual performance). Preparedness indicators thus fall into the following three categories:

Inputs are the constituent parts called for, implicitly or explicitly, by a given deliverable (personnel; standard operating procedures; equipment and supplies; or schedules of planned meetings, training, and other future activities).

Processes are evidence of actions taken to support or implement the plan (minutes of meetings, agreements prepared, training sessions conducted, or the numbers or percentages of personnel trained to use CBR agent detection equipment).

Outputs are evidence of the effectiveness of actions taken to support or implement the MMRS plan (establishment of a stockpile of antidotes and antibiotics appropriate for the agents that pose the greatest threat and demonstration of critical knowledge, skills, and abilities in tabletop exercises, full-scale drills, or surrogate incidents such as deliberate scares and false alarms, unintentional chemical releases, naturally occurring epidemics, or isolated cases of rare diseases).

The best evidence for preparedness will almost always be outputs, which are the end products of processes undertaken with inputs. A variety of circumstances, including the timing of the assessment, may make collection of output data impossible or impractical. In this circumstance, evidence for preparedness must be sought among inputs and processes. All three types of indicators are, however, merely surrogate or proxy measures of MMRS effectiveness that are based on the judgments of knowledgeable students of the field but that have never been truly validated (and that cannot be truly validated, short of an actual mass-casualty CBR terrorism incident). For each of the selected performance indicators, the committee then provided its opinion on what would constitute acceptable evidence of preparedness (preparedness criteria). Box ES-1 provides an example of one such indicator, with the associated criteria for preparedness, and Figure ES-1 shows the overall approach to analyzing preparedness.

The approach taken by the committee calls for a combination of evaluation of documents submitted to OEP by the community to be evaluated, direct observation of drills and exercises, and on-site questioning by a site-visit team. The indicator set therefore includes some components that may be evaluated through written materials, some that demand on-site questioning or observation, and some that can best be judged by observation of a community drill or exercise.

Exercises and Drills

The committee members began their task with the common view that, in the absence of regularly occurring CBR terrorism incidents, the plans produced by MMRS program cities might be best evaluated by large-scale field exercises that would simulate such an incident and more specialized drills that would test the performances of specialized portions of the overall response plan. This approach was ultimately rejected as too expensive in terms of the financial costs for OEP and in terms of time for local emergency response and medical personnel, difficult to tailor to 100 different locales, and in the case of a covert release of a biological agent, impossible to simulate realistically and ethically. Several committee members also observed that in their experiences the planning rather than the conduct of exercises had proven to be of greater value to the community.

Since one of the MMRS program contract deliverables in fact calls for a schedule of exercises and another calls for collection and distribution of after-action reports, the committee opted to incorporate these exercises into the overall evaluation plan. Observers, preferably members of the team that will subsequently conduct a site visit to the community in question, should attend large-scale exercises and significant drills before they

BOX ES-1
Example of Preparedness Indicator for One Essential Capability, First Responder Protection

Essential Capability

First Responder Protection

Preparedness Indicator

Demonstration that appropriate types and quantities of personal protective equipment and supplies have been purchased and are readily accessible to both traditional first responders and hospital and clinic staff.

Preparedness Criteria

- Amount and location of procured personal protective equipment are consistent with MMRS program planning document's presumed incident size and methodology for determining equipment needs.
- Inspection of at least two sites confirms the presence of equipment in specified inventory. Equipment should be readily accessible and clearly labeled at a site with appropriate temperature and humidity controls.
- Emergency and security staff have immediate access to personal protective equipment.
  - Equipment is stored in an area without a lock.
  - If it is stored in a locked area, staff can locate the key without assistance.
- On-duty personnel should be able to put on breathing apparatus (e.g., masks or respirators) without coaching. Respiratory fit test (e.g., with banana oil or peppermint oil) should confirm that the breathing apparatus seals completely.
- On-duty personnel should be able to put on chemical protective apparel without coaching. When suited, personnel should be heavily sprayed with water to demonstrate that the suit excludes outside elements (no water penetrates body suit).

plan a site visit. Despite the drawbacks mentioned in the previous paragraph, many of the essential capabilities can be more accurately analyzed in this fashion, and some can only be evaluated in this manner.

Site Visits and Peer Evaluators

Although the details of any site visit to some extent will be specific to the site being visited, the committee envisions a typical site visit consist-

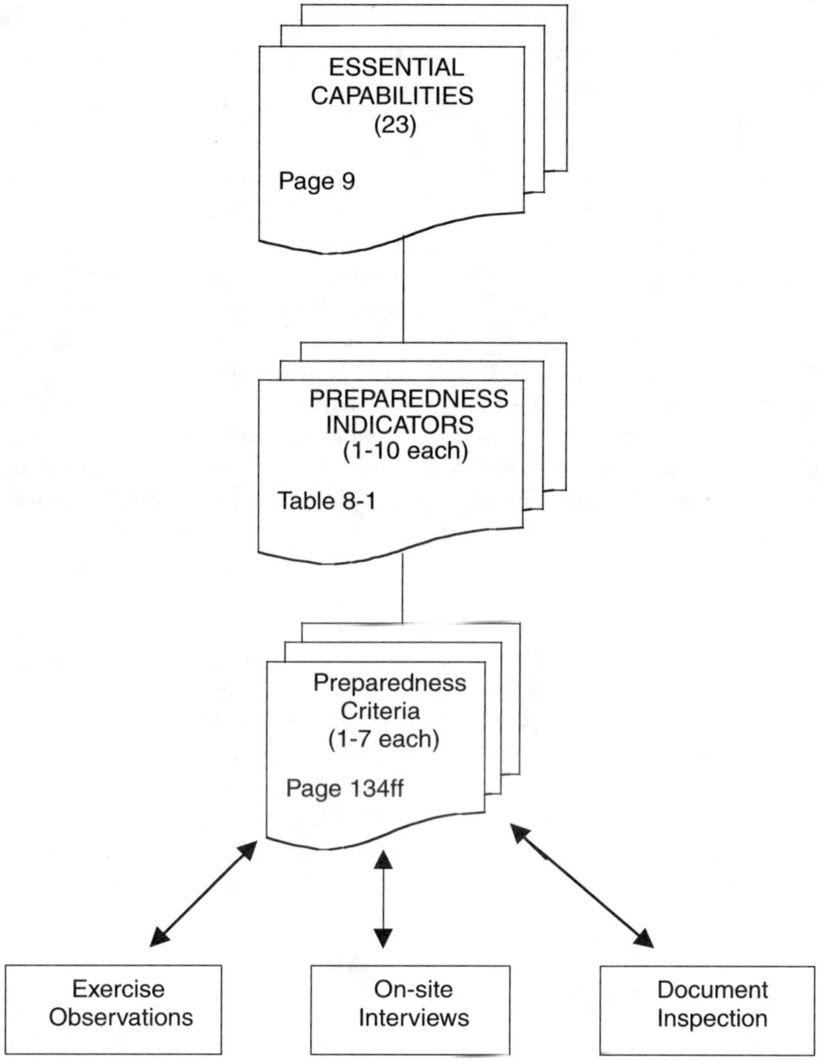

FIGURE ES-1 Relationships among essential capabilities, preparedness indicators, preparedness criteria, and data collection methods. All communities are evaluated for capabilities in 23 domains, the 23 essential capabilities listed above. Each capability is measured by reference to a set of 1 to 10 preparedness indicators (Table 8-1). For each preparedness indicator, evaluators draw a conclusion on preparedness based on the extent to which the community meets one to seven indicator-specific preparedness criteria (see Chapter 8). Data from the community are gathered by document inspection, on-site interviews, or observation of exercises and drills, as specified in the criteria.

ing of a 3-day evaluation that would include individual interviews and observations, two 3-hour scenario-driven group discussions that would take place simultaneously on the afternoon of Day 3, a briefing of the community (i.e., some very general feedback on the assessment team's observations and conclusions), and a formal report based on the collected observations of the assessment team.

The assessment team should consist of five individuals collectively experienced in a variety of disciplines and professions. They should be, and be perceived as, peers of the individuals being assessed. To this end the committee recommends a fire department representative familiar with hazmat operations; a city- or county-level emergency manager; a local public health officer familiar with surveillance systems; an individual with extensive managerial, operational, and clinical experience in the field of prehospital emergency medical services; and an acute-care medical practitioner, who could be a nurse or a physician, with clinical experience in infectious diseases or emergency medicine and mass-casualty operations. At least three of the five members should have some current or previous involvement with the MMRS in their own communities.

The scenario-driven group discussions, each facilitated by two on-site evaluators, will require 12 to 15 representatives from the community's safety and health institutions to discuss questions about the community's response to a fictional CBR terrorism incident. The goal of this portion of the site visit is to give the community an opportunity to demonstrate the existence of a well-understood process to coordinate all necessary capabilities to respond to a mass-casualty CBR terrorism incident, specifically the ability to acquire, process, and appropriately distribute information required to effectively manage critical incident functions. The fact that the evaluators will conduct two simultaneous discussions will insure that this ability is not confined to a single individual or a single department.

CLOSING REMARKS

The IOM committee's Phase I report suggested several activities or areas that might be useful additions to future contracts with additional cities (Institute of Medicine, 2001). Among these are a preliminary assessment of the community's strengths and weaknesses and provisions for the use and management of volunteers, for the receipt and distribution of materials from the National Pharmaceutical Stockpile, for decision making related to evacuation and disease containment, for the provision of shelters for people fleeing an area of real or perceived contamination, for postevent follow-up on the health of responders and caregivers, and for postevent amelioration of anxiety in the community at large. Nevertheless, the committee has been favorably impressed by the program's focus on empowering local communities, as opposed to creating yet another federal team to rush to the community at the time of an incident, and the program's flexibility in allowing each community to shape its system to its unique circumstances and requirements. A carefully done evaluation program of the sort described in this report should make the program even better.

Not only does it seem that the resources are now available for the continuing financial relationship suggested by the committee, but it also seems that a consensus now exists on the need for shared responsibility among a wide variety of governmental and nongovernmental agencies to achieve the goals of the MMRS program. When the committee began this project the future success of the MMRS program depended on voluntary cooperative efforts to prepare for possible but seemingly improbable events. As the project concludes, the committee believes that OEP must be empowered to take a stance that fosters voluntary collaboration but must be willing and able to enforce integration of local, state, and federal services as a pressing societal need for coping with inevitable future acts of terrorism.

The importance of the MMRS program effort is no longer equivocal, questionable, or debatable. The philosophy that it has developed has become an essential and rational approach that can be truly successful only with a rigorous and continuing evaluation and improvement program. The enhanced organization and cooperation demanded by a well-functioning MMRS program will permit a unified preparedness and public health system with immense potential for improved responses not only to a wide spectrum of terrorist acts but also to mass-casualty incidents of all varieties.

1

Introduction

In the wake of several major acts of terrorism in the early 1990s, some within the United States itself (the bombing of the Alfred P. Murrah Federal Building in Oklahoma City in 1995 and the World Trade Center bombing in 1993) and some in other countries (the release of nerve gas in the Tokyo subway in 1995), the U.S. federal government dramatically increased funding to combat terrorism. According to the Office of Management and Budget (2001), even before the awful events of September 11, 2001, more than $9.6 billion of the fiscal year 2001 federal budget was designated for such programs, including more than $1.7 billion for actions directed against terrorism with weapons of mass destruction (WMD), that is, nuclear weapons and chemical, biological, and radiological (CBR) agents. (The expenses incurred in responding to the results of the airliner hijackings on September 11, 2001, and to the effects of the mailing of the anthrax spore-laden letters that followed will undoubtedly add substantially to those totals when a full accounting is available.)

Among these federal efforts to combat terrorism with WMD is the Metropolitan Medical Response System (MMRS) program of the U.S. Department of Health and Human Services (DHHS), which attempts to enhance the preparedness of major U.S. cities to handle the health and medical consequences of an attack or threatened attack with CBR agents. That program is the subject of this report.

CHEMICAL, BIOLOGICAL, AND RADIOLOGICAL TERRORISM

CBR agents have become a focus of counterterrorism efforts because they possess a number of characteristics that would seem to make them attractive to terrorists. Dispersed via the air-handling system of a large public building, for example, a very small quantity of a CBR agent may produce as many casualties as a large truck full of conventional explosives, making the acquisition, storage, and transport of a powerful weapon much more feasible. Although not as easy to acquire or make as some have suggested, serviceable CBR weapons are within the intellectual, financial, and technological reach of many groups and individuals. Some CBR agents can be delivered very effectively as "invisible killers," that is, as colorless, odorless, and tasteless aerosols or gases, enhancing their psychological impacts and making it difficult to locate and identify the source. Some if not all CBR agents are also long-lasting threats. That is, contaminated victims of attacks with chemical, radiological, and some biological agents can spread the agent to others far from the scene of the initial release, and some infectious biological agents will ultimately transform the victims into carriers who can transmit the agent themselves. Lastly, the biological and radiological agents and some of the chemical agents of concern produce their deleterious effects only after delays of hours to days or weeks after exposure, facilitating the escape of the perpetrator and making detection of the attack difficult for both healthcare providers and law enforcement officials.

Chemical Agents

There are thousands of chemicals that at some dose may result in morbidity or mortality for humans. In the present context, "chemical agents" generally comprise a relatively short list of chemicals that at some time have been "weaponized" for military use. Some of these agents have no nonmilitary use (e.g., nerve agents and mustard gas); other agents such as chlorine and ammonia are widely used by industry. These agents are often classified by the site or nature of their effects in humans, such as nerve agents, blister agents, choking agents, vomiting agents, incapacitants, and tear agents; and many of these agents are not well known by civilian hazardous materials technicians and other emergency responders, medical personnel, or law enforcement officials. Even common industrial chemicals may be difficult to identify without specialized equipment when they are encountered in an unfamiliar context. The agents in Table 1-1 have been the primary focus of efforts to prepare for chemical terrorism, in part because of their toxicities but to a greater extent because of the health care community's unfamiliarity with these agents.

TABLE 1-1 Chemical Agents and Their Effects

Agent	Effects	Onset	First Aid
Nerve agents: tabun (GA), sarin (GB), soman (GD), GF, VX	Miosis, rhinorrhea, dyspnea, convulsions	Seconds to minutes	Decontamination, atropine, pralidoxime, ventilation, anticonvulsants
Vesicants (blister agents): mustard (H, HD), Lewisite (L), phosgene oxime (CX)	Erythema, blisters, eye irritation, blindness, dyspnea, coughing	Minutes to hours	Decontamination, topical antibiotics, bronchodilators, ventilation, British anti-Lewisite
Blood agents: hydrocyanic acid (AC), cyanogen chloride (CK), arsine, methyl isocyanate	Panting, convulsions, loss of consciousness, apnea	Minutes	Nitrites, sodium thiosulfate
Choking agents: phosgene (CG, DP), chlorine, ammonia	Tightness in the chest, coughing, dyspnea	Minutes to hours	Oxygen, bronchodilators, ventilation

SOURCE: Sidell et al. (1997).

Figure 1-1, taken from an earlier Institute of Medicine (IOM) publication (Institute of Medicine, 1999), illustrates in a very elementary way some of the actions required to cope with a chemical agent incident such as the one that took place in the Tokyo subway in 1995.

Biological Agents

Biological agents with adverse effects on human health include viruses, bacteria, fungi, and toxins. Specific toxins are included here rather than under chemical agents only because they are chemicals produced by a living entity (ricin from castor beans, saxitoxin from certain shellfish, and botulinum toxin from the bacterium *Clostridium botulinum*, for example). The distinguishing feature of biological agents other than toxins is their ability to propagate: exposure to an extremely small amount can lead to an overwhelming infection, and the victim may even become a source of infection for additional victims. This propagation within the exposed person (that is, incubation) takes time, however. The effects of viruses, bacteria, and fungi may not become apparent until days or weeks

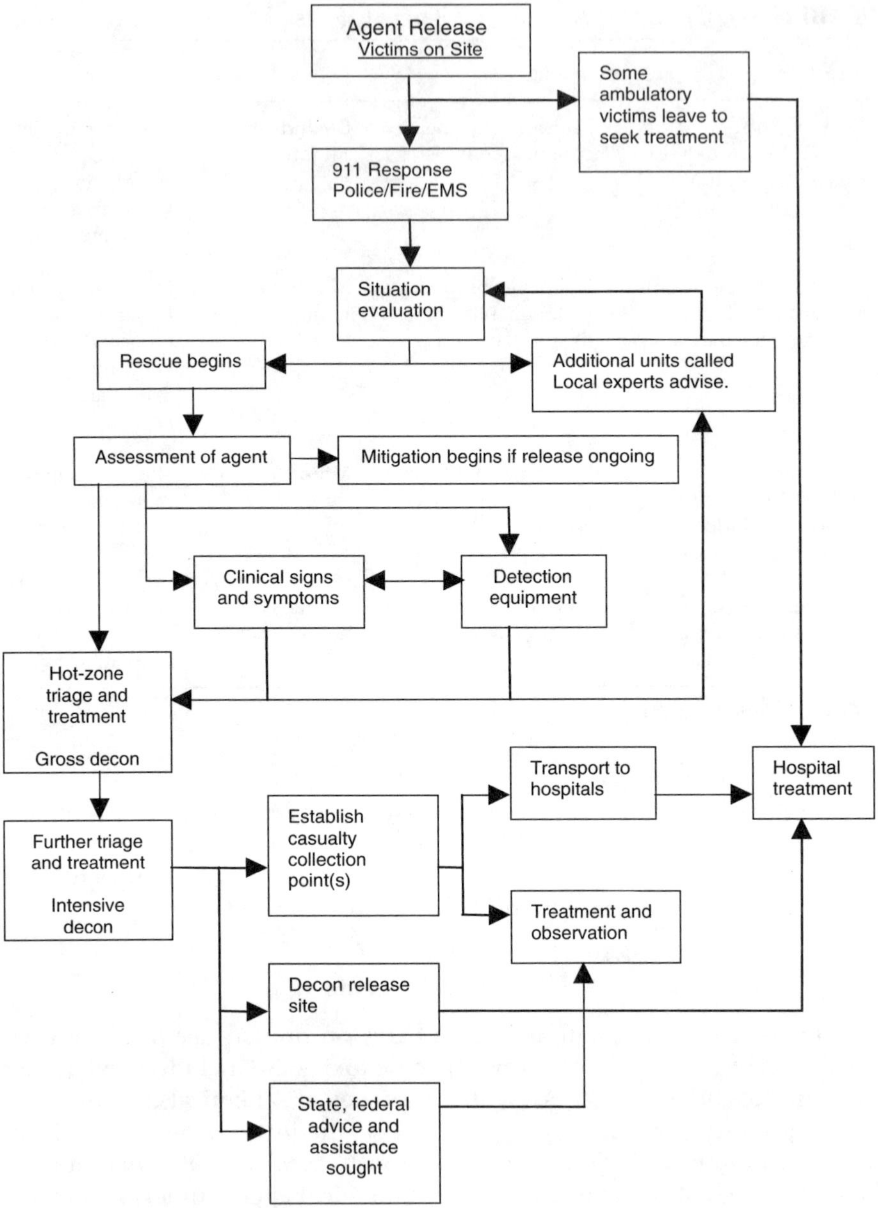

FIGURE 1-1 Flow chart of probable actions in a chemical or overt biological agent incident. EMS, emergency medical services; decon, decontamination. Source: Institute of Medicine (1999).

after the initial exposure, so there may be no obvious temporal or geographical concentration of victims to help medical personnel arrive at a diagnosis and make law enforcement personnel suspect a crime.

Diagnosis of the illness in individual patients will also be rendered more difficult because most of the agents considered to be likely threats are very rarely seen in U.S. cities and the initial symptoms that they produce (fever, headache, general malaise) are also characteristic of those produced by many common diseases. As difficult as it was to contain the spread of anthrax spores from just a few spore-filled letters in the autumn of 2001, the fact that the letters announced the presence of anthrax spores actually made the diagnosis and response far easier than if, for example, the perpetrator had covertly introduced spores into the air-handling system of a sports arena or airport. The victims in that case would have dispersed, perhaps very widely, by the time they became ill, and many might have died before an accurate diagnosis could have been made. Figure 1-2, from a previous IOM report (Institute of Medicine, 1999), illustrates some of the actions required to cope with the effects of a covert attack with a biological agent.

As in the case of chemicals, would-be terrorists have a very large number of potentially harmful biological agents from which to chose. Indeed, the tools of biotechnology might even be used to make some biological variants that have not previously existed, so to suggest that would-be terrorists will only use agents that have been the focus of military weapons programs would be folly. The agents that have been developed as biological weapons were carefully selected for their suitability as weapons, however, and few American physicians have experience in either the diagnosis or treatment of the diseases caused by those agents. For that reason, these agents have been the focus of counterterrorism training and other preparations. The specific agents that MMRS program cities are asked to consider in their planning are presented in Table 1-2 along with information on characteristics of the associated disease and on prophylaxis and treatment regimens currently recommended by the Centers for Disease Control and Prevention (CDC) and the U.S. Army Research Institute of Infectious Diseases..

Radiological Agents

The term "radiological weapon," in distinction to the term "nuclear weapon," refers to a weapon that would disseminate radioactive materials by means other than an uncontrolled fission chain reaction. The so-called dirty bomb, which consists of radioactive material wrapped around conventional explosives, is the best-known example. Nuclear power plants are the largest nonmilitary users of radioactive materials, but small

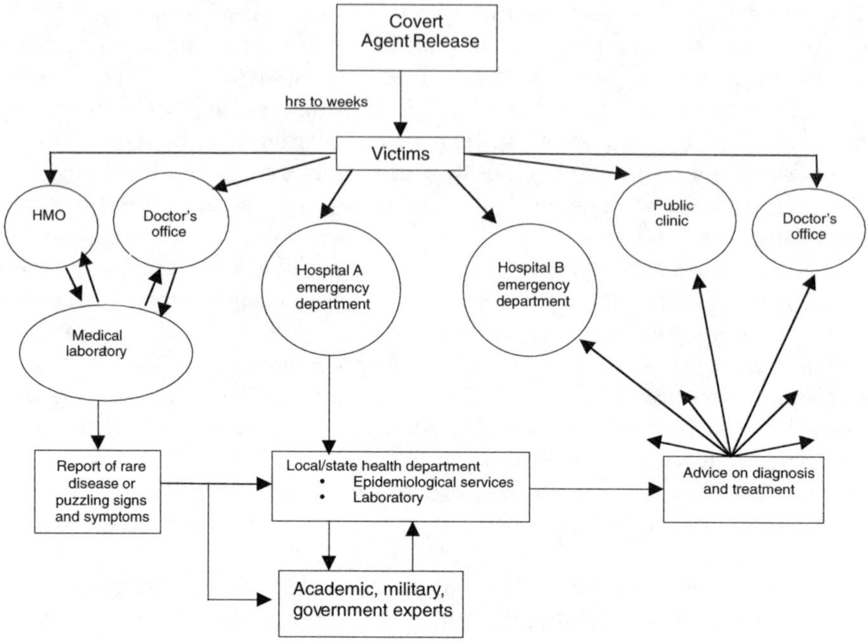

FIGURE 1-2 Flow chart of probable actions in a covert biological agent incident. HMO, health maintenance organization. Source: Institute of Medicine (1999).

quantities of radioactive materials are used in a variety of medical procedures at hundreds of locations throughout the United States. The radiation emitted in the decay of radioactive materials, as well as cosmic rays and conventional X rays, is called "ionizing radiation" because the radiation strips electrons from atoms and molecules that it encounters, including those in human tissue. Exposure to excessive amounts of ionizing radiation does not make one radioactive; but in the short run it can produce skin reddening and loss of hair, nausea and vomiting, diarrhea, sterility, tissue fibrosis, organ atrophy, bone marrow failure, and death. None of these effects are instantaneous, so radiological terrorism would present some of the same challenges for clinical diagnosis and law enforcement that covert bioterrorism would. Some of these effects may be temporary, but the genes of some exposed individuals may also be damaged, leading to cancer or birth defects in their offspring that are manifest only years later. No treatment other than symptomatic antinausea and antidiarrheal drugs is available for acute radiation sickness, but some evidence suggests that early intervention with potassium iodide can reduce the incidence of some long-term thyroid effects, especially in children (Verger et al., 2001; Zanzonico and Becker, 2000).

The rate of decay of the commonly used radioactive materials is very slow, so contamination is a serious clinical concern. Although not invisible, a finely ground or powdered agent could be detected and removed only with the aid of special detection equipment. Ionizing radiation comes in four forms, and although there are detectors for each of the four forms, no one piece of equipment on the market meets all detection requirements.

The activities required to cope with an incident involving a radiological weapon may resemble those outlined in either Figure 1-1 or Figure 1-2, depending on whether the attack is overt (perhaps a conventional bomb wrapped in highly radioactive material) or covert (introduction of radioactive dust into an air, water, or food supply).

THE MMRS PROGRAM

Today's MMRS program has evolved from an idea originally developed in the metropolitan Washington, D.C., area in 1995. Using the combined personnel and equipment resources from Washington, D.C., Arlington County in Virginia, and Montgomery and Prince Georges Counties in Maryland, the Metropolitan Medical Strike Team (MMST) received training, equipment, and supplies specifically designed to facilitate an effective response to a mass-casualty terrorism incident with a WMD. The first of its kind in the civilian environment, the MMST was designed to provide initial, on-site emergency health, medical, and mental health services after a terrorist incident involving CBR materials. The team's mission includes CBR agent detection and identification, patient decontamination, triage and medical treatment, emergency transportation of patients to local hospitals, coordination of movement of patients to more distant hospitals via the National Disaster Medical System, and planning for the disposition of nonsurvivors. Building from the initial efforts of the Washington Metropolitan Area MMST, the DHHS Office of Emergency Preparedness (OEP) funded the development of a similar team in Atlanta, Georgia, in preparation for the 1996 Summer Olympic Games.

The program expanded further when the U.S. Congress, as a part of the Defense Against Weapons of Mass Destruction Act of 1996, directed the Secretary of Defense to take immediate actions to both enhance the capability of the federal government to respond to terrorist incidents and to support improvements in the capabilities of state and local emergency response agencies. In recognition of this requirement, an amendment (widely known as the Nunn-Lugar II or Nunn-Lugar-Domenici Amendment, after its sponsors in the U.S. Senate) to the National Defense Authorization Act for Fiscal Year 1997 (P.L. 104-201) authorized $100 million to establish a military rapid response unit; to implement programs providing advice, training, and loan of equipment to state and local emergency

TABLE 1-2 Biological Agents, Effects, Characteristics, and Medical Countermeasures

Disease (Agent)	Effects of Inhalation	Incubation Period
Anthrax (*Bacillus anthracis*)	Fever, headache, fatigue, cough, dyspnea, death if untreated (the cutaneous form with black eschar has a much lower mortality rate)	1–5 days (up to 60 days possible)
Botulism[a] (*Clostridium botulinum* toxin)	Blurred vision, photophobia, difficulty speaking, progressive paralysis, respiratory failure, death	1–5 days
Brucellosis[b] (six species of the *Brucella* bacterium)	Fever, headache, chills, weakness, sweating, weight loss; seldom fatal	5–60 days
Hemorrhagic fever[a] (a dozen viruses from the families *Arenaviridae*, *Bunyaviridae*, *Filoviridae*, and *Flaviviridae*)	High fever, low blood pressure, subcutaneous hemorrhage, bleeding from mucous membranes, organ failure, death	4–21 days
Plague (*Yersinia pestis*)	Fever, chills, headache, nausea, vomiting, pneumonia and bloody sputum, septicemia, death	2–3 days
Smallpox (variola virus)	Fever, malaise, headache, backache, abdominal pain, rash, death in 20–30 percent of those exposed	7–17 days
Tularemia (*Francisella tularensis*)	Fever, weakness, prolonged weight loss; seldom fatal	2–10 days

[a]Added to MMRS program contracts beginning in 1999.
[b]Deleted from MMRS program contracts beginning in 1999.

response agencies; and *to provide assistance to major cities in establishing "medical strike teams"* (emphasis added).

This legislation provided funds in fiscal year 1997 for OEP to contract with the cities of Anchorage, Baltimore, Boston, Chicago, Columbus (OH), Dallas, Denver, Detroit, Honolulu, Houston, Indianapolis, Jacksonville, Kansas City (MO), Los Angeles, Memphis, Miami, Milwaukee, New York, Philadelphia, Phoenix, San Antonio, San Diego, San Francisco, San Jose, and Seattle. Similar appropriations in subsequent years allowed further

Communicability	Prophylaxis	Treatment
None; however, spores can survive for years outside the host	Preexposure: vaccine in use since 1960s Postexposure: oral antibiotics for 30 days plus vaccine or oral antibiotics for 60 days without vaccine	Inhalation: Intravenous antibiotics two times/day for 7 days and then orally for 53 days Cutaneous: oral antibiotics for 60 days
None	Vaccine available only through CDC	Supportive therapy; antitoxin available only through CDC
None	No vaccine approved	Oral antibiotics daily for 6 weeks
From patient fluids	Approved vaccine only for yellow fever	Supportive therapy, ribavirin for some viruses
Highly contagious via aerosol route	Preexposure: vaccine no longer available Postexposure: oral antibiotics for 7 days	Intravenous antibiotics twice daily for 14 days
Highly contagious via aerosol or contact with pustules	Vaccine is available only through CDC	Symptomatic treatment only
None	Postexposure: oral antibiotics for 14 days	Intravenous antibiotic for 7–21 days

SOURCES: Franz et al. (1997)), Institute of Medicine (1999), and Centers for Disease Control and Prevention (2001a,b).

expansion, and by Spring 2002, OEP had written contracts with 122 cities and was preparing to contract with 25 more.

Perhaps because the immediate stimulus for the program had been an incident in 1995 involving the release of a military nerve agent (sarin) in the Tokyo subway, the first two MMSTs were essentially enhanced hazardous materials (hazmat) teams; and their plans, training, and equipment centered around dealing with chemical agents. Some of the other early MMRS program cities changed the MMST concept by integrating strike team capabilities into existing fire department, emergency medical services, and police training and organizational infrastructures. In addition, their plans incorporated local public health officials; nongovernmental organizations; state agencies, including the National Guard; federal military and nonmilitary officials; and private health care organizations. OEP soon amended the initial contracts to focus more attention on coping with a covert release of a biological agent and changed the name of the program to the Metropolitan Medical Response System. The new name emphasizes that the program is intended to enhance the capabilities of existing systems that involve not just hazmat personnel, law enforcement personnel, emergency medical services personnel, public hospitals, and the American Red Cross but also public health agencies and laboratories, private hospitals, clinics, independent physicians, and other private-sector organizations. This emphasis on enhancing existing systems rather than creating new and perhaps competing, CBR weapon-specific systems was strongly recommended by a previous IOM committee as a first principle in efforts to prepare for CBR terrorism (Institute of Medicine, 1999).

The contracts between OEP and the MMRS program cities provide funds for special equipment and a cache of pharmaceuticals and medical supplies, and in turn demand detailed plans on how the city will organize and respond to chemical and biological terrorism incidents. A large number of these cities have now produced acceptable plans, and OEP turned to IOM for assistance in evaluating the extent to which its efforts and these plans have actually prepared cities to cope with the consequences of mass-casualty terrorism with a CBR agent (i.e., are the cities now well-prepared, and how has OEP contributed?). Specifically, OEP approached IOM about its ongoing need to a) systematically assess and evaluate the status of each MMRS program city (determining whether the program was having its intended effect of increasing preparedness) and b) understand the effectiveness of the overall program approach (determining whether OEP is doing an effective job of managing the program). Continuing improvement, as in any program, is critically dependent on regular evaluations of successes and shortcomings, a task rendered more difficult in this case by the low rate of actual incidents of terrorism involving CBR weapons.

CHARGE TO THE COMMITTEE

OEP charged the IOM Committee on Evaluation of the Metropolitan Medical Response System Program as follows:

> IOM shall identify and develop performance measures and systems to assess the effectiveness of, and to identify barriers related to, the MMRS development process. Additionally, IOM shall establish appro-

priate evaluation methods, tools, and processes, based upon the performance measures, to assess the MMRS development process.

In Phase I, an expert committee shall identify, recommend, and develop performance measures and systems to assess the effectiveness of, and identify barriers related to, the MMRS development process at the site, jurisdictional, and governmental levels. When developing the performance measures the contractor should include the following:

a. How can OEP measure, at the program level, whether the strategies, resources, mechanisms, technical assistance, and monitoring processes provided to the MMRS development process are effective?

b. How can OEP identify whether the performance objectives identified in the MMRS contract lead communities to preparedness?

c. What modifications, additions, and/or subtractions should be made to these performance objectives to assist communities throughout the development process?

d. How can existing standards be used to validate these performance objectives? If standards do not exist, how can new standards be created and/or the performance objectives be validated?

e. What strategies have communities used to enhance their existing capabilities? What are the most effective means to measure these additional capabilities?

f. Can relationships between traditional first responders/public safety officials and their supporting hospitals/public health offices be assessed? If so, how?

g. What tools and/or models exist to measure preparedness for natural disasters?

h. Do current federal performance measures for natural disasters or other programs (mitigation and response) have application to WMD terrorism preparedness (e.g., Project IMPACT)?

i. How can casualty assumptions, for communities of varying populations, be established (percentage of population, historical data)?

j. How can OEP measure the preexisting systems, methodologies, and plans that are used by public safety, public health, and health services agencies to communicate during day-to-day operations? How can OEP measure the impact that the MMRS development process has had on the level and/or expectations for this communication?

k. How can financial barriers related to WMD preparedness be identified and measured?

In Phase II, the committee shall use the performance measures developed from Phase I to recommend and then develop appropriate evaluation methods, tools, and processes to assess the MMRS development process. When developing these methods, tools, and processes the committee should, at a minimum, address the following:

a. What is the most appropriate approach/model to evaluate the MMRS development process (e.g., surveys, interviews, review of plans, peer review, operational tests, etc.)?
b. Is there an appropriate sample size that would adequately represent the impact of the MMRS development process?
c. Considering the variance in local health systems, how can OEP appropriately draw meaningful conclusions from the results of this evaluation?

The evaluation system(s) developed should be geared toward the timely assessment of each deliverable or phase of the development process with emphasis placed on identifying barriers, identifying solutions, and sharing successes of both the technical and administrative components of the MMRS program.

A Phase I report delivered to the sponsor in October 2001 (Institute of Medicine, 2001) provided some initial observations on the program and its management, answered the specific questions posed by OEP for consideration during Phase I of the project. Because the primary measure of effectiveness for any program is the extent to which it achieves its ultimate goals, the Committee also identified almost 500 preparedness indicators that might be used to assess the response capabilities of MMRS program cities at the site, jurisdictional, and governmental levels. Those indicators are described in the committee's Phase I report (Institute of Medicine, 2001) and are reprinted here in Appendix E. In Phase II, the committee used the preparedness indicators established in Phase I to develop usable evaluation methods, tools, and processes for assessing both program management by OEP and the capabilities of the local communities necessary for effective response to CBR terrorism. Those methods, tools, and processes are the subject of this second and final report.

METHODS OF THE PRESENT IOM STUDY

In the autumn of 2000, IOM assembled a committee whose members provided expertise in the fields of emergency medicine, emergency and disaster management, urban planning, epidemiology, public safety, public health, hospital administration, infectious diseases, mental health services, and program evaluation. This was accomplished in accordance with the established procedures of the National Academies, including an examination of possible biases and conflicts of interest and the provision of an opportunity for public comment. Brief biographies of each of the committee members are provided in Appendix A.

The committee used a wide variety of sources to assemble the data and information necessary to respond to its charge. An initial organizational and data-gathering meeting of the committee in December 2000 provided an overview of the MMRS program from the viewpoints of both OEP and several of the initial MMRS program cities. Other speakers provided an overview of program evaluation principles and practices and some insights into two Federal Emergency Management Agency (FEMA) programs focused on assessing state and local readiness for a variety of potential disasters. At a subsequent meeting, in February 2001, the committee learned details of the legislative and executive origins of the MMRS program and other federal counterterrorism programs. At that same meeting representatives from the U.S. Department of Justice and the Centers for Disease Control and Prevention described their current programs aimed at enhancing state and local capabilities, and a Public Health Service project officer described the different approaches and levels of success achieved by the 16 MMRS program cities in his geographic area. In addition, that meeting also featured briefings on the assessment techniques and procedures used by medical organizations evaluating residency programs, poison control centers, and individual physician specialists and by FEMA's National Urban Search and Rescue Team program. Discussions with the speakers provided more detailed information and points of contact for additional questions.

As additional sources of information, the sponsor's project officers shared file copies of completed plans from six MMRS program cities and offered committee members contacts and resources in the OEP offices that had relevant data. The committee members themselves contributed both personal contacts and specific information from their own files and experience. The World Wide Web provided much information about additional organizations and training in counterterrorism; and the committee staff assembled a library of more than 500 documents, published and unpublished, bearing on federal, state, and local preparations for managing the consequences of a terrorist incident involving a CBR weapon.[1]

An interim Phase I report, released in October 2001, was the result of extensive discussion among the committee members at a 2-day meeting in May 2001 during which the committee drafted answers to each of the specific questions asked by OEP in its charge to the committee and compiled initial preparedness indicators. Subsequent revisions of the preparedness indicators were reviewed and modified via email, and committee members signed off on the review draft in late July 2001. After review

[1]These documents and other written materials presented to the committee are maintained by the Public Access Office of the National Research Council Library. Appointments to view these materials may be made by telephoning the library at (202) 334-3543 or by sending an e-mail to nrclib@nas.edu.

by a panel of nine independent reviewers and attendant revisions to the manuscript, the Phase I report was released in October 2001 (Institute of Medicine, 2001). A similar process, with meetings held in October 2001 and January 2002, led to the present report.

ORGANIZATION OF THIS REPORT

Following this introductory chapter, Chapter 2 describes emergency response systems, local, state, and federal, and how the MMRS program fits into those activities.[2] Chapter 3 describes federal programs other than the MMRS program that aim at proactively strengthening state and local capabilities to respond to CBR terrorism. Chapter 4 describes the details of the contracts between OEP and the MMRS program cities that define the program. Chapter 5 provides an overview of evaluation concepts and introduces some principles for application to the MMRS program. Chapter 6 describes the committee's derivation of nearly 500 potential preparedness indicators (the indicators themselves are provided in Appendix E). Chapter 7 addresses OEP's management of the program by providing OEP with a self-report instrument with which to query MMRS program communities about their perceptions of the MMRS program and OEP's administration of the program. Chapter 8 addresses the effectiveness of the program itself. It draws on a subset of the preparedness indicators to describe the committee's recommendations for a three-part program for assessing the capabilities of the MMRS program communities. Finally, Chapter 9 presents a brief summary and the committee's overall conclusions and recommendations for improving the MMRS program. Appendixes provide brief biographies of the committee and staff, descriptions of federal teams available to respond to the scene of terrorism involving a CBR agent, a list of MMRS program cities, the checklist with which OEP evaluates MMRS contract compliance, a collection of nearly 500 preparedness indicators potentially applicable to the MMRS program that was the product of phase I of this IOM project, and fictional biological, chemical, and radiological scenarios with discussion questions.

---

[2]The committee is indebted to Lauren Schiff for a commissioned paper that was the basis for Chapter 2.

2

Community Emergency Management and Available Federal Assistance

A previous Institute of Medicine (IOM) study (Institute of Medicine, 1999) pointed out that despite the justifiable emphasis on the novel aspects of a possible terrorist attack with a chemical or biological agent, frameworks for responding to incidents of both types already exist. An attack with a chemical agent would be similar to the hazardous materials incidents that metropolitan safety personnel confront regularly; a major mission of public health departments is the prompt identification and suppression of infectious disease outbreaks; and poison control centers deal with poisonings from both chemical and biological sources on a daily basis. In addition, most major metropolitan areas have, and are occasionally called upon to use, plans to cope with natural disasters that could result in a large number of casualties. As the IOM report emphasized,

> It would be a serious tactical and strategic mistake to ignore (and possibly undermine) these mechanisms in efforts to improve the response of the medical community to additional, albeit very dangerous, toxic materials. Strengthening existing mechanisms for dealing with unintentional releases of hazardous chemicals, for monitoring food safety, and for detecting and responding to infectious disease outbreaks is preferable to building a new system focused solely on potentially devastating but low-probability terrorist events. Indeed, a major reason for the committee's decision to focus the report on response to aerosol attacks with the short list of agents thought to be a threat by U.S. military forces was that these agents are unfamiliar to the U.S. civilian medical system. Regardless of relative probability of use or relative lethality, there are mechanisms in

> place for dealing with a wide variety of other agents and routes. Our concern was not to foster construction of yet another mechanism, but to encourage the incorporation of these unfamiliar agents and routes into existing mechanisms (Institute of Medicine, 1999, p. 185).

This chapter briefly describes those existing mechanisms for dealing with emergencies and disasters other than chemical, biological, and radiological (CBR) terrorism; delineates four other federal programs aimed at improving state and local capabilities to deal with CBR terrorism; and thus, puts the Metropolitan Medical Response System (MMRS) program into a larger perspective.

EMERGENCY MANAGEMENT TERMINOLOGY

To understand modern emergency management, it is important to first describe the terminology used to define hazards, the magnitudes of emergencies, and management activities. Communities in the United States face a variety of hazards that can cause loss of life and injury, property damage, and significant economic consequences. A *hazard*, in its simplest definition, is a condition or event with the potential to cause harm to the community or environment (Federal Emergency Management Agency, 1997b). Three categories of hazards can be distinguished: natural, technological, and conflict (Sylves, 1998). *Natural hazards* are phenomena brought about by "nature," including tornadoes, earthquakes, floods, volcanoes, fires, severe storms, temperature extremes, and disease. *Technological hazards* (also referred to as man-made or human-caused hazards) include aircraft crashes, plant explosions, and hazardous materials incidents. Recently, a third category, *conflict hazard*, has been used to distinguish human-caused incidents that involve intentional destruction of life or property. They include war, terrorism, civil unrest, and riots. These categories can be used to define the initial cause of a disaster, but they are not always mutually exclusive. For example, a small flash flood may damage a chemical plant and cause a massive hazardous material release. This is a case of a natural hazard triggering an even greater technological hazard.

Hazards of comparable magnitude can cause very different amounts of damage. To continue with the flash flood example, if the flood were to enter a rural area, it may require an immediate response by public safety and medical personnel. This event would be defined as an *emergency*, an unexpected event that jeopardizes life or property and that requires an immediate response through the use of available community resources and procedures (Drabek, 1996). If this same flood were to enter a crowded, industrial area, it could overwhelm the local community's capacity to respond and recover, requiring additional resources from outside agencies. A *disaster* is defined as a calamity beyond the coping capacity of the affected population, whether triggered by natural or technological hazards or by human action (Disaster and Emergency Reference Center, 1998) A *major disaster* causes "damage of sufficient severity and magnitude to warrant major disaster assistance under the Robert T. Stafford Disaster Relief and Emergency Assistance Act (42 U.S.C. § 5121 et seq. [1974]) to supplement the efforts and available resources of states, local governments, and disaster relief organizations in alleviating the damage, loss, hardship, or suffering caused thereby" (Federal Emergency Management Agency, 1999a).

Human impact depends not only upon the magnitude of the hazard but also its evolution. Earthquakes, tornadoes, and explosions, for example, occur suddenly and without warning, whereas temperature extremes and infectious diseases generally have a slower and even insidious onset. All hazards, however, are addressed through four basic phases of emergency management: mitigation, preparedness, response, and recovery. *Mitigation* activities are designed to alleviate the effects of a major disaster or emergency or to minimize the potentially adverse effects of those that are unavoidable (Federal Emergency Management Agency, 1996a, 2000b). This may include enforcing building codes and developing safety regulations. *Preparedness* encompasses activities, programs, and systems that exist before an emergency and that are used to prepare people to respond appropriately or bolster resources for effective response (Federal Emergency Management Agency, 2002a). Preparedness includes evacuation and hardening of buildings, short-term activities that can be performed to lessen damage before a disaster. *Response* is defined as activities that address the immediate and short-term effects of an emergency or disaster. Response includes immediate actions to save lives, protect property, and meet basic human needs (Federal Emergency Management Agency, 1999b). Finally, *recovery* consists of long-term activities and programs that occur beyond the initial crisis period of an emergency or disaster and that are designed to restore systems to normal status or to rebuild them in a less vulnerable condition (Federal Emergency Management Agency, 1996b). These phases occur cyclically within a community; for example, a community that has just recovered from a recent hurricane may begin mitigation projects to protect itself against the next one.

Although disasters are not new, several trends are cause for concern: the costs of disasters are rising as increases in populations and rates of development occur in hazard-prone areas, technological disasters are also on the rise as a result of the development of new industries and the aging of the existing infrastructure, and conflict hazards have become increasingly menacing. The field of emergency management is evolving to minimize the growing impacts of disasters.

EMERGENCY MANAGEMENT IN THE UNITED STATES

Emergency management is the management of personnel and complex systems to address hazards and their impacts through the four phases described above. It is a rapidly evolving profession and therefore is not practiced in a uniform manner throughout the United States. Within the last century, a number of emergency services have emerged to save lives and prevent property damage, including emergency medical, fire, police, and public health services. The coordination of these services has its roots in wartime civil defense measures but has evolved to cover a broader spectrum of resources and emergencies. The Federal Emergency Management Agency (FEMA) defines emergency management as "organized analysis, planning, decision-making, and assignment of available resources to mitigate (lessen the effect of or prevent), prepare for, respond to, and recover from the effects of all hazards. The goal of emergency management is to save lives, prevent injuries, and protect property and the environment if an emergency occurs" (Federal Emergency Management Agency, 1995, p. 3). Today, emergency management also includes mitigation to build disaster-resistant communities.

By definition, a "system" is a set of interrelated parts working together to achieve a common goal. The goal of the emergency management system is to reduce the loss of life, property, and environmental damage through the close coordination and cooperation of people, organizations, and resources. As stated by researcher Richard Sylves, "No single agency can manage a disaster effectively. In the American system, the response effort requires the resources and expertise of law enforcement, the fire service, emergency medical personnel, public health and public works people, and many others" (Sylves, 1998, p. 145). These parts must work together in a coordinated manner, each understanding their roles "so that they can effectively use resources and aid disaster victims" (Sylves, 1998, p. 145).

The importance of the systems approach is reflected in an important concept in U.S. emergency management: "all-hazards" management. In the past, localities developed individual plans for each type of hazard, with separate mechanisms to respond to each. A community would have separate plans for tornadoes, flooding, severe storms, nuclear emergencies, and industrial explosions. Emergency management professionals have recognized that a range of management functions is common to all incidents and that the availability of a *single set of systems* for managing emergency responses is advantageous and is the basis for the all-hazards approach to emergency management. For example, the function of warning is necessary in every emergency so that people will understand, trust, and respond appropriately to the message, regardless of the type of hazard. Similarly, incident management, patient tracking, health surveillance, information management, and restoration of lifeline services are common functions that are addressable through a common and consistent system.

By recognizing that multiple hazards can be responded to with a single set of management and response systems, communities benefit from cross-training, increased efficiency, and avoidance of duplication. The process of developing an all-hazards plan also promotes coordination across organizations, prevents conflicts in planning, and avoids gaps in disaster response. Emergency management formulated on the basis of multiple hazards also promotes flexibility and an increased ability to respond to the unexpected. Concurrently, practitioners of the all-hazards approach must recognize that disasters may vary in terms of their predictability, duration, speed of onset, magnitude, scope, and impact and in terms of the possibility of secondary impacts. Special actions (such as radiation monitoring) may also be required for specific hazards.

In the United States, emergency management follows a bottom-up approach; its core is at the local jurisdiction, with supplementation and assistance from outside resources as necessary. The immediate post-impact response relies heavily on local emergency service personnel and other resources from the affected community, which networks to provide essential aid. This network often involves volunteers, businesses, media, nonprofit organizations, and academia. As the size or complexity of an event increases or as the event crosses local boundaries, resources may be acquired from outside the local jurisdiction, often from higher levels of government. The first level of assistance comes from regional resources; neighboring local governments often develop mutual-aid agreements to fill special needs or combine resources to aid a locality in a time of crisis. Many large incidents affect areas across local (and often state) jurisdictional boundaries, requiring response assistance throughout metropolitan areas for adequate management. (For the purpose of this chapter, metropolitan areas will be referred to generically as regions.)

If the event threatens to overwhelm the resources of a region or requires specialized assistance, the role of the state increases to provide resources and to serve as a conduit to the federal level. Federal emergency management primarily provides aid through the states. This assistance is not intended to supersede or replace activities at lower levels but is instead intended to supplement these activities.

Bottom-up emergency management is a result of the U.S. federalist system in which sovereignty is shared among multiple levels of government. Although the federal government provides national legislation and executive direction, it is the direct responsibility of the local and state political jurisdictions to protect their residents and provide emergency services. Historically, no federal disaster response force has the authority to assume control and manage emergency operations unless local responsibility has been abdicated. The U.S. disaster response architecture therefore evolved to one based upon shared authority and decentralization of responsibilities. The involvement of numerous resources with shared responsibility demands close coordination and cooperation among multiple levels of government and among the general public, business and industry, and nonprofit organizations.

LOCAL EMERGENCY MANAGEMENT

Emergency management efforts at the city or county level begin long before an incident with the implementation of mitigation measures such as enforcement of building codes, careful land management, development of written emergency response plans, creation of an emergency response structure, and other community investment to reduce vulnerabilities and preparation for hazards. At the outset of an incident, emergency managers are directly involved in coordinating personnel and resources for response, usually from an emergency operations center, where multiple city departments work together. It is the local public safety organizations (police and fire departments, emergency medical services [EMS], public works departments, and others) that will be the first on scene for sudden emergencies and that will arrive within the most critical time frame for saving lives and protecting property. Local and regional medical and public health personnel will also be rapidly involved and will very likely be the first to notice atypical symptoms and developing trends among the victims of hazards involving infectious disease agents or insidious toxins. Local leaders are the ones who understand both local priorities and the consequences of critical decisions. During the recovery period, it is the local jurisdiction that will be performing the rebuilding long after additional resources have dispersed.

The response to the 1995 bombing in Oklahoma City illustrates the practice of a local jurisdiction that provided immediate resources and whose efforts were supplemented, but not supplanted, by state and federal resources. On April 19, 1995, the Alfred P. Murrah Federal Building was the target of a massive terrorist bomb. The Murrah Building partially collapsed, and many surrounding structures were severely damaged by the explosion. The Oklahoma City Fire Department (OCFD) responded to the scene to provide immediate rescue efforts, established incident command, and coordinated the interagency response throughout the disaster under a local incident commander (Marrs, 1995).

A total of 759 people were injured or killed in the blast (Mallonee et al., 1996). Health and medical issues were handled by a number of organizations at all levels of government and private business that all reported to the same command system. Emergency Medical Services Authority, a private ambulance service, transported victims to hospitals. Fire, emergency medical, and police departments in surrounding areas provided mutual aid by performing services at the bombing site and by responding to baseline emergencies in other areas of the jurisdiction while city resources were busy at the scene. The state medical examiner's office tracked missing persons, identified recovered victims, and notified families. The state office of emergency services interfaced with the FEMA urban search-and-rescue teams, which assisted OCFD with the rescue of victims and the recovery of bodies.

Local, state, and federal resources provided security on the scene and carried out investigations. The Oklahoma City Police Department (OCPD) established perimeters, identified the evidence recovery area, and maintained control of the surrounding streets. OCPD worked with the Federal Bureau of Investigation (FBI) in the recovery of evidence and criminal investigations and directed state and federal military personnel resources. Public works personnel were essential to scene safety and maintenance; they cut off electric power and natural gas to affected buildings, established sanitary facilities for rescue workers and lighting for nighttime operations, and picked up refuse. The local telephone company installed an emergency cellular phone system to assist with communications. Fire, police, EMS, and other resources from surrounding jurisdictions responded through preestablished mutual-aid agreements to assist at the scene and to cover public safety functions in areas of Oklahoma City unaffected by the bombing (Marrs, 1995).

The OCFD incident commander attributed much of the success of the response to the emergency training that personnel of all city departments received and to an effective incident management structure. Investment in adequate training and other preparedness measures can be a significant obstacle for communities, however. Disasters are low-probability, high-consequence events, meaning that they occur infrequently, but when they do occur their effects are devastating. The infrequency of disasters often makes it difficult for communities to justify spending on emergency management when faced with seemingly more urgent and ongoing public needs. Once a disaster occurs, funding for response and recovery activities can be substantiated because the needs are apparent. Preparation and mitigation measures, which could save many more lives and cost much less, often become "back-burner" issues, as the funding needs are not as obvious. Potential funding is also limited by the fact that local governments are "at the end of the line" for pass-through federal and state emergency management funding (National Academy of Public Administration, 1993).

One result of such funding decisions is that local jurisdictions often focus primarily on hazards that are most threatening to their area or develop capabilities to meet their most recent event. For example, cities in California may be very well prepared for earthquakes, cities in the Midwest have warning systems and procedures that specifically deal with tornadoes, and cities along the East Coast have designed emergency systems such as evacuation procedures around the threat of hurricanes. Although they are prepared for their highest-probability hazards, communities in these regions are often not well prepared to respond to other, less expected hazards.

Communities that have strong systems in place rather than resources directed primarily at specific hazards, conversely, can respond better to unexpected events. This is especially true in hazardous materials incidents when responders must often deal not only with unknown substances but also unknown combinations of substances. In July 2001, a 60-car freight train derailed in a 1.5-mile-long tunnel near the heart of Baltimore, Maryland. The train was carrying several containers of hazardous materials, some of which ignited an extremely hot fire. The incident triggered a response from five fire departments; shortly thereafter, a hazardous materials task force was also called in from South Baltimore. The disaster was complex because the responders were combating a mixture of multiple hazardous materials; in addition, the fire was located in a confined space, but smoke and liquid runoff affected a wide area (Kiehl and Niedowski, 2001). To protect public health and safety, Baltimore police shut down area roads, including interstate highways and the U.S. Coast Guard blocked access to portions of Baltimore's Inner Harbor. Health officials monitored air quality, and members of the Baltimore Fire Department went door to door to warn residents to shelter in place and keep windows closed (Layton and Phillips, 2001).

This incident resulted in no deaths because the teams were prepared with appropriate training and equipment. A formal command system that enabled decision makers to make informed and coordinated judgments about the health and safety of the responders and the community was also established. The coordination of information must extend beyond the incident command system to instruct the public on appropriate actions. These difficulties will also be present in a large-scale chemical terrorism event if an MMRS program is not successfully developed.

It is especially important for emergency public health and medical systems to be well integrated with local and regional emergency management systems so that measures to protect public health are appropriate and timely. In the summer of 1995, several heat waves hit Chicago, Illinois, posing a subtle yet extremely serious hazard to public health. Chicago implemented a plan to provide air-conditioned shelters. Shelters went unoccupied, however, as elderly individuals perished in their homes because of their reluctance to leave, a lack of access to transportation, or a lack of knowledge of the services that were available. The city recognized this problem and revised its plan. During a second heat wave several days later, the city dispatched city workers to knock on the doors of elderly individuals to deliver food and water and to provide transportation to the cooling shelters (Terry, 1995).

Coordination between local and state public health departments, physicians, and emergency management officials was also key in the West Nile virus outbreak in New York City in 1999 (Fine and Layton, 2001; Nash et al., 2001). During that year, the West Nile virus killed seven people and infected numerous others in the New York City area. This virus had never before been seen in the United States, and the response of New York City to this outbreak shows how the public health system operates to detect and respond to disease outbreaks, regardless of the source. In this case, a physician in Queens noticed a pattern of unusual symptoms in two patients and, because encephalitis is a reportable condition in New York City, contacted the New York City Department of Public Health. which immediately began a search for possible additional cases at area hospitals. Six more cases were identified in Queens within a week, and initial laboratory tests by the New York State Department of Health and the Centers for Disease Control and Prevention (CDC) suggested a flavivirus infection. The symptoms of the patients were consistent with a diagnosis of St. Louis encephalitis (SLE), which is not uncommon along the Eastern seaboard. SLE is known to be transmitted by *Culex* mosquitos, so mosquito control measures were immediately begun in the area affected by the outbreak. These included aerial spraying, distribution of mosquito repellent, door-to-door searches for potential mosquito breeding sites, and a major public education effort.

A final piece of the puzzle fell into place when public health officials learned that zoo and veterinary experts were conducting another investigation of unusual deaths among birds in the same area. Flaviviruses were not thought to kill birds, but the fact that many of the dead birds showed evidence of viral encephalitis suggested that the two outbreaks might be related nonetheless. Four weeks after the recognition of the outbreak in humans a flavivirus later identified as West Nile virus was isolated from tissue of crows and a flamingo in a local zoo and subsequently determined to be the common cause of both the avian and human disease outbreaks. West Nile virus is transmitted by *Culex* mosquitos, just as SLE is, and no additional cases had occurred in the Queens area where mosquito control measures had been initiated. The fact that avian cases had been observed over a much larger range led to both additional case-seeking in all 72 New York City hospitals and a massive expansion of the mosquito control effort.

A September 2000 study of New York City's response to the West Nile virus outbreak found that this communication and coordination between responding agencies was a key lesson that could be applied to public health preparedness for bioterrorism (U.S. General Accounting Office, 2000a). The study noted, however, that although the system worked, there were several obvious places for improvement. A single alert physician at a local hospital initiated the investigation early enough that an effective intervention was possible before the outbreak became a disaster, but the investigation subsequently found many other cases which were either not properly diagnosed or not reported to the health department. Much more systematic surveillance and reporting at the local level is needed. Similarly, improved communication among public health agencies, including those dealing with animal health, is needed. Increased laboratory capacity will also be important to an efficient and effective response to disease outbreaks (only one public health laboratory in the country was initially equipped to diagnose West Nile virus).

STATE ASSISTANCE

Local jurisdictions request state assistance to obtain specialized resources, to supplement local resources, or to act as a financial or operational conduit to federal resources. State governors have the legal responsibility to carry out emergency preparedness, response, and recovery actions; and declaration of an emergency provides him or her with additional powers. These powers include the authority to mobilize the National Guard, to order an evacuation, to commandeer and use private property (within prescribed limits), to use emergency funds, and to enter into mutual-aid agreements with other states.

Every state has an emergency management office, but the organization and proximity of that office to the governor vary widely. Ten states have emergency management agencies at the cabinet level within the office of the governor. Beauchesne (2001) reported that 22 states have emergency management functions within the department of military affairs and that 12 others have such functions within departments of public safety. The remainder of states structure emergency management functions within combined public safety-military affairs agencies, within community or local affairs departments, or within the state police department. During nonemergency periods, the role of the state is to develop emergency management programs that complement and promote local emergency management capabilities. The state has the legal authority to enact codes and regulations and to enforce state and national laws (Sylves, 1998). The state emergency management office often maintains the state emergency management plan, an emergency operations center, and services that are activated upon local request for assistance.

The National Academy of Public Administration observes that the states are in a unique position to gauge the emergency management needs of more than one of its political subdivisions, assess its own and to some extent the federal government's resources, and facilitate the acquisition and application of these resources (National Academy of Public Administration, 1993). State agencies are responsible for coordination of emergency services, horizontally with other states (for mutual assistance) and vertically when federal resources are necessary, for the state often serves as the conduit between local and federal governments. The Emergency Management Assistance Compact provides a framework for coordinating interstate assistance (Emergency Management Assistance Compact, 2002), whereas the federal response plan's concept of operations details the framework for requesting and managing federal assets (Federal Emergency Management Agency, 1992).

Some states provide assistance for a wide variety of emergencies; others have responsibilities and resources only for certain types of incidents (Beauchesne, 2001). These services may include the provision of specialized resources (e.g., search-and-rescue teams and hazardous materials technicians), emergency management training, or management assistance. States have very different approaches and devote different resources to emergency management. California employs approximately 800 people in its Office of Emergency Services (OES). The California OES is located within the governor's office and is well funded to provide Internet-based systems to coordinate and manage state disaster responses, response equipment (including 120 state-owned fire engines), and, among many other services, a fully staffed training institute for emergency management. California not only provides resources but also has a strong hand in responses to emergencies and events through the coordination of mutual aid within the state (California Office of Emergency Services, 2002). Maryland, on the other hand, operates a 40-person emergency management agency within the Maryland Military Department. The Maryland Emergency Management Agency operates an emergency operations center on an as-needed basis, coordinates federal programs, and organizes a rapid response team consisting of 13 state organizations frequently involved in disaster response (Maryland Emergency Management Agency, 2002).

THE FEDERAL EMERGENCY RESPONSE PLAN

When the demands of disasters exceed local, regional, and state capabilities, the federal government is called upon to provide supplemental assistance. If needed, the federal government can mobilize an array of resources to support state and local efforts. Various emergency teams, support personnel, specialized equipment, operating facilities, financial assistance programs, and the provision of access to private-sector resources constitute the overall federal disaster operations system.

Under the Robert T. Stafford Disaster Relief and Emergency Assistance Act (42 U.S.C. § 5121 et seq. [1974]), a governor may request the President to declare a major disaster or an emergency if an event is beyond the combined response capabilities of the state and the local governments that are affected. If an emergency involves an area or facility for which the federal government exercises exclusive or primary responsibility and authority, the President may unilaterally direct the provision of emergency assistance under the Stafford Act. The governor of the affected state will be consulted if possible.

Federal assistance takes many forms—including the direct provision of goods and services, financial assistance (through insurance, grants, loans, and direct payments), and technical assistance—and can come from various sources. Initial sources include internal government supplies (available surplus and excess property or agency stock previously acquired from the Disaster Relief Fund or on hand). Agencies also may acquire needed goods and supplies from outside the federal government, such as from the private sector and possibly nonaffected state and local governments. FEMA has been given responsibility for coordinating, planning, and managing this assistance, a task that it carries out in accordance with the Federal Response Plan (FRP) (Federal Emergency Management Agency, 1992).

The FRP describes the policies, planning assumptions, concept of operations, response and recovery actions, and responsibilities of 27 federal departments and agencies and the American Red Cross that guide federal operations following a presidential declaration of a major disaster or emergency. The FRP uses a functional approach that groups under 12 emergency support functions (ESFs) the types of direct federal assistance that a state is most likely to need (e.g., mass-casualty care or health and medical services), as well as the kinds of federal operational support necessary to sustain a federal response (e.g., transportation and communications support). Each ESF is headed by a primary agency designated on the basis of its authorities, resources, and capabilities in the particular functional area. The 12 ESFs are

1. transportation,
2. communications,
3. public works and engineering,
4. firefighting,
5. information and planning,
6. mass care,
7. resource support,
8. health and medical services,
9. urban search and rescue,
10. hazardous materials,
11. food, and
12. energy.

Emergency Support Function 8, Health and Medical Services

The U.S. Department of Health and Human Services (DHHS) is the lead federal agency with responsibility for ESF 8, health and medical services. In that role DHHS coordinates the provision of federal health and medical assistance to fulfill the requirements identified by the affected state and local authorities. Included in ESF 8 are the overall public health response; triage, treatment, and transportation of victims of the disaster; and evacuation of patients out of the disaster area. Resources for this aid come from the following:

- within DHHS;
- ESF 8 support agencies (e.g., the U.S. Department of Defense [DOD], the U.S. Department of Transportation, the American Red Cross, and the Environmental Protection Agency [EPA]);
- the National Disaster Medical System (NDMS), a nationwide medical mutual-aid network between the federal and nonfederal sectors that provides patient evacuation and definitive medical care; at the federal level, it is a partnership between DHHS, DOD, the U.S. Department of Veterans Affairs (VA), and FEMA; and
- specific nonfederal sources such as major pharmaceutical suppliers, hospital supply vendors, the National Foundation for Mortuary Care, certain international disaster response organizations, and international health organizations.

ESF 8 describes 15 specific functional areas of federal health and medical assistance, as follows:

1. Assessment of health and medical needs. DHHS deploys an assessment team to the disaster area to assist in determining the specific

health and medical needs and priorities. This function includes the assessment of the infrastructure of the health care system and health care facilities.

2. Health surveillance. CDC helps establish surveillance systems to monitor the general population and special high-risk segments of the population, carry out field studies and investigations, monitor injury and disease patterns and potential disease outbreaks, and provide technical assistance and consultations on disease and injury prevention and precautions.

3. Medical care personnel. The Office of Emergency Preparedness (OEP) provides Disaster Medical Assistance Teams (DMATs) and individual public health and medical personnel to assist in providing care for ill or injured victims at the location of a disaster or emergency. DMATs can provide triage, medical and surgical stabilization, and continued monitoring and care of patients until they can be evacuated to locations where they will receive definitive medical care. Specialty DMATs can also be deployed to address burn injuries, pediatric care requirements, chemical injury or contamination, and so forth. In addition to DMATs, active-duty and reserve military units and National Guard units with casualty clearing-casualty staging and other missions are deployed as needed. Individual clinical health care and medical care specialists may be provided to assist state and local personnel. VA is one of the primary sources of these specialists.

4. Health and medical care equipment and supplies. OEP provides health and medical care equipment and supplies, including pharmaceuticals, biological products, and blood and blood products, in support of DMAT operations and for the restocking of health and medical care facilities in an area affected by a major disaster or emergency.

5. Patient evacuation. OEP, through NDMS, moves seriously ill or injured patients from the area affected by a major disaster or emergency to locations where definitive medical care is available. NDMS patient movement will primarily be accomplished with the fixed-wing aeromedical evacuation resources of DOD.

6. In-hospital care. OEP, through NDMS, provides definitive medical care to victims who become seriously ill or injured as a result of a major disaster or emergency. For this purpose, NDMS has established and maintains a nationwide network of voluntarily precommitted, federal and nonfederal acute-care hospital beds in the largest U.S. metropolitan areas.

7. Food, drug, and medical device safety. The Food and Drug Administration ensures the safety and efficacy of regulated foods, drugs, biological products, and medical devices following a major disaster or emergency. It also arranges for the seizure, removal, and destruction of contaminated or unsafe products.

8. Worker health and safety. CDC assists with monitoring the health and well-being of emergency workers, performs field investigations and studies addressing worker health and safety issues, and provides technical assistance and consultation on worker health and safety measures and precautions.

9. Radiological, chemical, and biological hazards consultation. CDC assists with assessing the health and medical effects of radiological,[1] chemical, and biological exposures on the general population and on high-risk population groups; conducts field investigations, including collection and analysis of relevant samples; provides advice on protective actions that can be taken to prevent direct human and animal exposure and indirect exposure through radiologically, chemically, or biologically contaminated food, drugs, water supplies, and other media; and provides technical assistance and consultations on medical treatment and decontamination of radiologically, chemically, or biologically injured or contaminated victims.

10. Mental health care. The Substance Abuse and Mental Health Services Administration assists in assessing mental health needs; provides disaster-related mental health training materials for disaster workers; and provides liaisons with the assessment, training, and program development activities undertaken by federal, state, and local mental health officials.

11. Public health information. CDC assists by providing public health and disease and injury prevention information that can be transmitted to members of the general public who are located in or near areas affected by a major disaster or emergency.

12. Vector control. CDC assists with assessing the threat of vector-borne diseases after a major disaster or emergency; conducts field investigations, including the collection and laboratory analysis of relevant samples; provides vector control equipment and supplies; and provides technical assistance and consultation on protective actions regarding vector-borne diseases and the medical treatment of victims of vector-borne diseases.

13. Potable water and disposal of wastewater and solid waste. The Indian Health Service assists in assessing potable water and issues related to the disposal of wastewater and solid waste; conducts field investiga-

[1]The lead agency and federal response to a radiological emergency will be based on the type or amount of radioactive material involved, the location of the emergency, the impact on or the potential for an impact on the public and environment, and the size of the affected area. The Federal Radiological Emergency Response Plan spells out the roles of federal agencies and takes precedence over the FRP.

tions, including collection and laboratory analysis of relevant samples; provides water purification and wastewater and solid-waste disposal equipment and supplies; and provides technical assistance and consultation on potable water and issues related to the disposal of wastewater and solid waste.

14. Victim identification and mortuary services. OEP and NDMS assist by providing victim identification and mortuary services, including NDMS Disaster Mortuary Teams; temporary morgue facilities; victim identification by fingerprinting, forensic dental, molecular biology, and forensic pathology-anthropology methods; and processing, preparation, and disposal of remains.

15. Veterinary services. OEP and NDMS assist in delivering health care to injured or abandoned animals and performing veterinary preventive medicine activities after a major disaster or emergency, including conducting field investigations and providing technical assistance and consultation as required.

In 1995, Presidential Decision Directive 39 (PDD-39), U.S. Policy on Counterterrorism, was issued to "establish policy to reduce the Nation's vulnerability to terrorism, deter and respond to terrorism, and strengthen capabilities to detect, prevent, defeat, and manage the consequences of terrorist use of weapons of mass destruction (WMD)" (Federal Emergency Management Agency, 1999b, p. 1). Approximately 2 years later, FEMA created the Terrorism Incident Annex to the FRP to describe the roles of federal agencies in responding to the consequences of terrorism within the United States. The annex defines two phases of the response to terrorism that may overlap: crisis management and consequence management. As described in the FRP Terrorism Incident Annex, *crisis management* "refers to measures to identify, acquire, and plan the use of resources needed to anticipate, prevent, and/or resolve a threat or act of terrorism" (Federal Emergency Management Agency, 1999b, p. 1). Crisis management is defined as a federal responsibility, predominantly involving law enforcement activities, with state and local assistance as appropriate. The FRP Terrorism Annex describes *consequence management* as "measures to protect public health and safety, restore essential government services, and provide emergency relief to governments, businesses, and individuals affected by the consequences of terrorism" (p. 1). As opposed to crisis management, consequence management is the responsibility of state and local governments, with support from the federal level as needed (Federal Emergency Management Agency, 1999b).

The Chemical and Biological Appendix to ESF 8

In recognition of some of the distinctive features of a major act of domestic terrorism with chemical or biological agents, DHHS has formulated an appendix to the ESF 8 section of the FRP specifying the federal government's response to urgent health and medical care needs resulting from such acts (U.S. Department of Health and Human Services, 1996). This support plan identifies 20 specific, specialized, and time-sensitive health and medical services functions, in addition to the 15 identified in ESF 8 proper; assigns responsibility for the response to each of those 20 functions to federal departments, agencies, and offices; and describes some of the assets available for the responses required. It carefully notes that any or all of the plan may be activated before a presidentially declared disaster to save lives and that the need for rapid action demands that some elements of the plan be organized and prepositioned ahead of any terrorist event.

Whether DHHS is assisting the FBI in evaluating a threat or responding to requests for assistance from FEMA and the affected community after an actual release of a chemical or biological agent, the special contributions of DHHS deal with threat assessment, emergency consultation, and specialized technical assistance. One of the first actions to be undertaken by DHHS after telephonic or electronic consultation would be deployment of an interagency Chemical and Biological Rapid Deployment Team of 23 technical specialists from DHHS, DOD, the U.S. Department of Energy, and EPA. Since the appendix was written, OEP has equipped and trained four specialized National Medical Response Teams (NMRT) to provide medical care for victims of weapons of mass destruction. Like the 23 DMATs, the NMRT can deploy to disaster sites within 12 to 24 hours and sustain themselves for a period of 72 hours while providing medical care at a fixed or temporary medical care site.

THE NATIONAL CONTINGENCY PLAN

The National Oil and Hazardous Substances Contingency Plan (also known as the National Contingency Plan [NCP]) is the plan for the federal response to oil spills and the release of hazardous substances. This plan outlines the National Response System for the reporting, containment, and cleanup of spills. It also established regional and national reaction teams and a response headquarters. Originally published in 1968, NCP was broadened several times to remain current with new legislation. It now covers hazardous-substance spills, oil discharges, and emergency removal actions for hazardous waste sites (Environmental Protection Agency, 1999). In the event of a spill, the plan is immediately activated, requiring no request from state or local levels; up to 16 federal agencies led by EPA and the U.S. Coast Guard may be involved, depending on the expertise and resources required.

THE FEDERAL RADIOLOGICAL EMERGENCY RESPONSE PLAN

After the Three Mile Island nuclear power plant accident in 1979, the lead role in offsite planning for radiological emergencies was transferred from the U.S. Nuclear Regulatory Commission (NRC) to FEMA. On-site activities continue to be the responsibility of NRC. Today FEMA is the federal lead for all types of peacetime radiological emergencies; through its Radiological Emergency Preparedness (REP) program, the agency works to ensure the health and safety of residents near nuclear power plants and to educate the public about radiological emergency preparedness. The REP program includes regional assistance committees, which assist with the development of state and local plans, and the Federal Radiological Preparedness Coordinating Committee, which issues policy and guidance on emergency response plans and procedures with the assistance of additional federal agencies (Federal Emergency Management Agency, 2000c).

The Federal Radiological Emergency Response Plan provides the framework for the federal response to peacetime radiological emergencies (Federal Emergency Management Agency, 2002c). State and local agencies are responsible for the measures needed to protect life and property in facilities and areas that are not controlled by the federal government (e.g., private reactors). However, they can request assistance directly from the federal agencies that are a part of the Federal Radiological Emergency Response Plan. All costs are the responsibility of the participating agencies.

TERRORISM-SPECIFIC FEDERAL SUPPORT TEAMS

In addition to the DMATs and related teams that constitute part of the DHHS response to a request for support from a community or communities suffering a catastrophic terrorist incident, a myriad of teams from other agencies are prepared to respond. Figure 2-1, taken from a September 2001 review of federal assets for combating terrorism conducted by the U.S. General Accounting Office (GAO), shows only the key consequence management teams (U.S. General Accounting Office, 2001a). Appendix B, from a slightly earlier GAO report (U.S. General Accounting Office, 2000b), provides selected information on the capabilities of many of those teams.

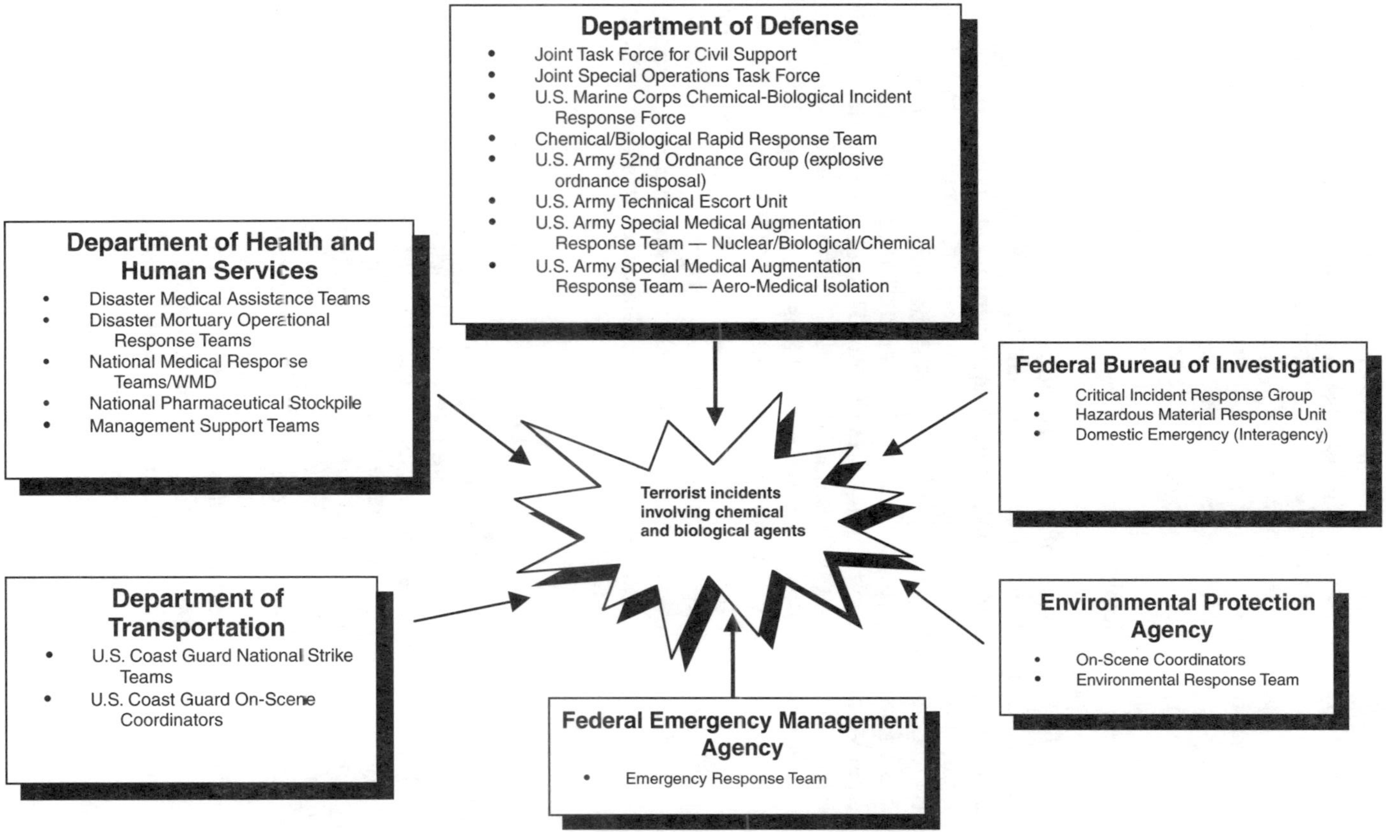

FIGURE 2-1 Key federal consequence management response teams for CBR terrorism (U.S. General Accounting Office, 2001a).

GAO (U.S. General Accounting Office, 2000b) and several high-level advisory groups (Advisory Panel to Assess Domestic Response Capabilities for Terrorism Involving Weapons of Mass Destruction, 2000; Cilluffo et al., 2000; Rudman, 2001) have repeatedly pointed out the need for better coordination among the many agencies with antiterrorism or counterterrorism programs. Terrorism is both a crime and a national security issue, so an array of crisis management teams and personnel, headed by the FBI, may also arrive at the scene, with or without a request from local law enforcement officials.

In May 2001 President George W. Bush reinforced the position of FEMA as the coordinator of federal responses to acts of domestic terrorism by establishing the Office of National Preparedness in that agency and charging it with coordinating and implementing all federal programs providing relief or support to local governments responding to acts of terrorism. Under this plan, the FBI remained the leader of criminal investigations of acts of terrorism, but in October 2001 President Bush signed an executive order establishing the Office of Homeland Security within the Executive Office of the President (Bush, 2001) and named Tom Ridge, a former governor of Pennsylvania, to head it as Assistant to the President for Homeland Security. The mission of the Office of Homeland Security is to develop and coordinate the implementation of a comprehensive national strategy to secure the United States from terrorist threats or attacks, including coordinating the executive branch's efforts to detect, prepare for, prevent, protect against, respond to, and recover from terrorist attacks within the United States.

CONCLUSION

The focus of this report is on planning and preparation for a terrorist attack in local communities before a terrorist attack occurs. However, it should be clear from this brief review of the federal resources available to assist with the consequence management of a completed act of terrorism that planning conducted before an incident occurs must address not only when and how to obtain federal help but also how to accommodate and coordinate that help upon its arrival. In this case, it is clearly possible to receive too much of a good thing. Nevertheless, it would be reasonable to conclude from the information presented in this chapter that the larger metropolitan areas of the United States have initiated substantial preparations for CBR terrorism, have in place some well-developed systems for coping with mass-casualty incidents of many sorts, have practiced the use of those systems, and have access to a large number and a wide variety of specialized federal resources. The next chapter reviews the much smaller number of federal programs aimed specifically at helping state and local authorities better adapt their systems to respond to the specific threats posed by CBR weapons.

3

Federal Efforts to Increase State and Local Preparedness for Terrorism

The preceding chapter's review of the Federal Response Plan makes it clear that the federal government is prepared to provide a substantial amount of diverse forms of assistance to communities stricken by a disaster. However, by even the most optimistic projections of the federal agencies themselves, none of this assistance will be available to the affected community until at least 12 to 24 hours after it is requested (and the request itself may not come for hours or even days after the initiating event, be it an earthquake, a flood, or the release of a chemical, biological, or radiological [CBR] agent). One of the distinguishing features of the Metropolitan Medical Response System (MMRS) program is that it is proactive. It is not just a new or better way of providing federal aid to stricken communities, but it is a way to help the communities themselves deal both with the initial stages of the disaster and with the subsequent influx of outside assistance. The MMRS program provides predisaster assistance; it is not a federal response. Chapter 4 provides details of the program, which provides funds for the purchase of special CBR agent-specific equipment, supplies, and pharmaceuticals for local law enforcement, fire department, and emergency medical personnel, but the program demands substantial integrated planning by the local partners. An important element of that planning involves knowledge of at least four other federal entities that provide additional equipment and CBR agent-specific training. These entities are the U.S. Department of Justice's (DOJ's) Office of Domestic Preparedness (ODP; formerly the Office of State and Local Domestic Preparedness Support [OSLDPS]), the Federal

Bureau of Investigation (FBI), the Centers for Disease Control and Prevention (CDC), and the Federal Emergency Management Agency (FEMA).

ODP PROGRAMS

As noted in Chapter 1, the Nunn-Lugar-Domenici Amendment to the National Defense Authorization Act for Fiscal Year 1997 (P.L. 104-201) designated the U.S. Department of Defense (DOD) as the head of an interagency program to assist civilian officials at all levels of government to better prepare for possible terrorist attacks with weapons of mass destruction (WMD). The law also gave the President the option of transferring responsibility for this "domestic preparedness" program to another agency any time after October 1, 1999, an option exercised by President Clinton in fiscal year 2000 by making DOJ the lead agency. DOJ was chosen at least in part because under the aegis of Title VIII of the Anti-Terrorism and Effective Death Penalty Act of 1996 (P.L. 104-32), DOJ, in conjunction with FEMA, had already begun a program to provide a 16-hour basic awareness course for fire and emergency medical services personnel through the National Fire Academy. DOJ assumed responsibility for this training in 1998 under P.L. 105-119 and organized OSLDPS to assist state and local response agencies (most often police and fire departments) in five interrelated areas: funding for special equipment, training, technical assistance, assessment, and exercise support. OSLDPS was renamed ODP in 2001.

Equipment

Grants of up to $300,000 are available for purchase of personal protective equipment (for example, chemical protective clothing and respirators), devices for field detection or identification of radioactive materials or selected military chemical or biological agents, equipment for mass decontamination of personnel or equipment, and communications equipment. In accordance with congressional direction, applications for these funds were initially taken from the 157 most populous metropolitan areas (unlike DOD and the U.S. Department of Health and Human Services [DHHS], which focused on the most populous core cities, DOJ used the Census Bureau's most populous "metropolitan statistical areas," 96 of which are counties rather than cities). All but a dozen of these jurisdictions have received training and associated equipment, and when the remainder of the 157 have been accommodated, DOJ will provide grants only to states and only contingent upon the state's preparation of two documents for DOJ : a statewide needs assessment and a 3-year domestic preparedness strategy. These documents, developed in conjunction with city, county, and other local jurisdiction emergency, health, and law enforcement agencies, will then guide both DOJ and the states in distributing the grant money to the appropriate agencies (U.S. Department of Justice, 2002a).

Training

Under the ODP emergency response training initiative, training courses are developed and delivered through a variety of venues and are directed at a broad spectrum of emergency responders, including fire, hazardous materials (hazmat), law enforcement, emergency medical services, public health, emergency management, and public works agencies (U.S. Department of Justice, 2002b).

ODP draws upon a large number of resources to develop and deliver these training programs, including private contractors, emergency response organizations, the National Domestic Preparedness Consortium (NDPC), and other agencies from the local, state, and federal levels. All training and course materials are free to eligible jurisdictions, as determined by ODP, but to attend a training class delivered by one of the ODP training partners, a request must be provided to the designated training point of contact. The courses, the duration of which varies from several hours to 5 days, cover CBR materials at four levels:

- *awareness-level* courses, which are designed for the entry-level first responder to gain basic knowledge of agents of WMD and safe response practices;
- *operations-level* training, which is designed for those students who have a firm grasp of basic responses and who seek to further their knowledge of incidents involving WMD;
- *technician-level* training, which is designed for students who are well versed in all levels of the response to the use of a WMD and which uses practical knowledge through hands-on training and exercises; and
- *command-level* modules, which are designed for senior-level incident management personnel who have a strong background in coordinating emergency responses.

All courses are described in a comprehensive on-line catalog (U.S. Department of Justice, 2002e).

ODP's course Emergency Response to Terrorism: Basic Concepts is available for on-site delivery to interested fire service and emergency medical services agencies. A limited number of positions may also be available for law enforcement personnel. This 2-day program is available as simple instruction, as a train-the-trainer course, or as a self-study course. The training provided through this course is available at no cost, and more than 50,000 individuals have taken the course.

ODP provides technical training in the handling of the equipment purchased through ODP programs that provide grants for the purchase of that equipment. This training is available upon the jurisdiction's request either through on-site visits or long-distance learning or at training facilities around the country, including the Equipment Training Center at Pine Bluff Arsenal in Arkansas.

Perhaps the centerpiece of DOJ training is the Center for Domestic Preparedness (CDP) in Anniston, Alabama, at the former Fort McClellan home of the U.S. Army's Chemical Defense Training Facility. CDP is one of only two facilities in the United States where individuals can be trained in a contaminated environment by use of live agents (actual chemical warfare agents). Three 4-day courses are offered: WMD Specialist, WMD Advanced Operations, and WMD Command. Travel, meals, lodging, and training are provided at no cost to the organization or responder, but CDP trains only about 200 responders a month, and there is a waiting list for each of the three courses (a 60- to 90-day wait is about average).

Other courses are available through NDPC, a partnership among DOJ, DOE, and three public universities. The courses provide training and run exercises on the operational and technical aspects of responding to terrorism involving WMD at its complex of consortium facilities, through regional courses, and via distance-learning technology. The National Energetic Materials Research and Testing Center of the New Mexico Institute of Mining and Technology provides field exercises and training with live explosives. The National Center for Bio-Medical Research and Training at Louisiana State University supplies training in biological agents and law enforcement. The National Emergency Response and Rescue Training Center at Texas A&M University specializes in training and field exercises on urban search-and-rescue techniques. The National Exercise, Test, and Training Center at the Nevada Test Site conducts large-scale field exercises using live agents, simulations, and explosives.

Technical Assistance

ODP provides free technical assistance of three types to state and local jurisdictions that request it. (1) General technical assistance provides assistance in such areas as development of a plan for responding to the use of a WMD and development and evaluation of exercise scenarios. (2) Technical assistance with state-level strategies helps states complete the required needs and threat assessments (see the next section on assessment) and the 3-year strategy that follows from them. (3) Equipment-related technical assistance provides training on the calibration, use, and maintenance of specialized equipment used to respond to the release of CBR agents.

Assessment

As noted in the section above on equipment, ODP has created and supplied to each state's designated administrative agency a multipart needs assessment that must be completed and returned as a prerequisite for the future receipt of equipment and training grants (U.S. Department of Justice, 2002c). The document instructs the state agency to gather data from all local jurisdictions with self-report forms and to then consolidate them into a document for the entire state. The forms include instruments developed by the FBI and the CDC to evaluate vulnerabilities, threats, and the performance of the public health sector. These are combined with assessments of required and current capabilities in the realms of fire services, hazmat services, emergency medical services, law enforcement, public works, public health, and emergency management. A 100-page "Tool Kit" is provided for use by the state and local personnel assigned to fill out the forms.

Exercises

As part of DOJ's first responder training and domestic preparedness initiative, the conference report (U.S. House of Representatives, 1998b) accompanying the act providing appropriations to DOJ for fiscal year 1999 provides $3.5 million for situational exercises for state and local emergency response personnel. The language of the conference report further directs that a portion of these funds be used to comply with language found in the Senate report (U.S. Senate, 1998), which discusses two types of exercises. The first is a major national-level TOPOFF exercise involving TOP OFFicials from federal, state, and local governments. The other incorporates situational exercises as part of DOJ's efforts to improve the capabilities of state and local emergency response personnel to incidents of domestic terrorism. Similar language is found in the House report (U.S. House of Representatives, 1998a, p. 13), which directs that the use of "confidence building exercises based on threat driven scenarios" be incorporated into DOJ's training efforts. The 10-day TOPOFF exercise, which featured a simulated biological agent incident in Denver, Colorado, and a simultaneous chemical weapons incident in Portsmouth, New Hampshire, took place in May 2000.

In addition to its National Exercise and State and Local Domestic Preparedness Exercise Programs, ODP, in collaboration with the U.S. Department of Energy (DOE), is establishing the Center for Exercise Excellence at the Nevada Test Site. The Center for Exercise Excellence plans to deliver a Weapons of Mass Destruction Exercise Training Program for the nation's emergency response community to ensure nationwide operational consistency in exercises related to incidents involving a WMD (U.S. Department of Justice, 2002d).

FBI PROGRAMS

The FBI is the lead federal agency responsible for crisis management, which includes "measures to identify, acquire, and plan the use of resources needed to anticipate, prevent, and/or resolve a threat or act of terrorism." (Federal Emergency Management Agency, 1999b, p. 1). It employs almost 1,400 agents in counterterrorism activities, including WMD coordinators in 56 field offices whose responsibilities explicitly include antiterrorism and counterterrorism activities. Within the FBI, the two primary offices that support state and local domestic preparedness are the National Domestic Preparedness Office (NDPO) and the Hazardous Devices School (HDS).

National Domestic Preparedness Office

NDPO does not provide direct assistance to state and local jurisdictions; instead, it serves as an information clearinghouse for state and local agencies on all aspects of domestic preparedness and coordinates federal policy regarding the provision of assistance with domestic preparedness to state and local jurisdictions (National Domestic Preparedness Office, 2002). In concert with those roles, NDPO is actually an interagency office, even though it is housed in FBI headquarters and is funded by the FBI. Representatives from DOD, DOE, the Environmental Protection Agency (EPA), FEMA, FBI, DHHS, the National Guard Bureau, the Nuclear Regulatory Commission, DOJ, and the U.S. Coast Guard, along with state and local experts from a variety of disciplines, form the NDPO staff. The State and Local Advisory Group provides additional input.

NDPO provides services in the following areas:

- Training. NDPO maintains a compendium of federal training courses in WMD and coordinates the establishment of emergency response training standards.
- Equipment. NDPO attempts to coordinate federal efforts to provide state and local governments with equipment for the detection of WMD, protection from WMD, and decontamination after the use of a WMD.
- Exercises. NDPO assembles a database of after-action reports from

federal, state, and local exercises, scenario templates, and other resources for state and local use.

- Planning. NDPO provides emergency responders access to federal, state, and local preparedness plans in the event of the use of a WMD.
- Information sharing. NDPO uses the Internet to provide information to the emergency response community on a wide variety of topics and formats, including a monthly newsletter, a secure network for emergency responders, and a toll-free help line.

Most or all of these missions and services are scheduled to be transferred to the Office of Homeland Defense and FEMA in 2002.

Hazardous Devices School

Located at Redstone Arsenal in Alabama, the Hazardous Devices School (HDS) trains public safety personnel in technology used to render explosive devices safe and offers the only national certification program for state and local bomb technicians (Federal Bureau of Investigation, 2000). In 1998, the school developed a 1-week WMD-related emergency action course and integrated this training into its standard course in 1999. By July 2000, more than 2,000 bomb technicians, virtually all of the certified bomb technicians in the United States, had received the training. HDS also manages the State and Local Bomb Technician Equipment Program, which provides protective, diagnostic, and detection equipment to the roughly 435 state and local bomb squads that have received or that are in the process of receiving accreditation from the FBI.

CDC PROGRAMS

CDC's Bioterrorism Preparedness and Response Program coordinates the efforts of eight different CDC offices and centers aimed at enhancing state and local capabilities to detect and respond to bioterrorism (Lillibridge, 2001). Unlike the DOJ and DOD programs, which primarily focus on fire and law enforcement actions in a chemical incident, the CDC programs target the public health infrastructure, that is, state health departments and local health departments, and terrorism involving biological agents. In fiscal year 2000, CDC devoted $155 million and 100 people to this effort in four core areas: pharmaceutical stockpiles, state and local capacities, CDC capacity, and independent studies.

The National Pharmaceutical Stockpile involves rapid-response "push packages" that contain a wide variety of pharmaceuticals and other medical materials to control outbreaks of infectious diseases and other emergencies, plus a vendor-managed inventory (VMI) of the same materials.

Unlike the push packages, which are standardized packages that sacrifice specificity for speed, the VMI can supply large quantities of incident-specific supplies, albeit not so quickly. Governors, but not mayors, can make requests directly to CDC for supplies from either component.

The push packages, located at 12 sites throughout the United States, are prepackaged collections ready for deployment anywhere in the United States via ground or air transportation in 12 hours or less. A single push package fills a Boeing 747 or seven 48-foot tractor-trailers and can treat 340,000 patients for 10 days. Supplies and equipment for repackaging of the pharmaceuticals are included, but everything comes in bulk form. CDC advisers accompany it; but the state is required to provide trucks, forklifts, security, personnel, electrical power, climate-controlled storage space, refrigerated storage space, and one or more licensed pharmacists to break down the package into single-dose-sized units and distribute them to health care providers.

During the anthrax attacks from October 15 to November 29, 2001, CDC used the VMI instead of the push packages to provide antibiotics since the infectious agent was known and anthrax-specific shipments could be assembled. The NPS program accomplished this in response to 65 requests from 10 different states and the District of Columbia and provided treatment or prophylaxis for more than 30,000 Americans.

One way in which state and local infrastructures are being strengthened is by the development of a national laboratory network to respond to bioterrorism. CDC now has dedicated laboratory space and rapid turnaround procedures to test for all six agents on its critical biological agents list; but more importantly, 72 state public health laboratories in 50 states now have some capacity to test for plague, tularemia, and anthrax, and 22 state public health laboratories can test for botulinum toxins.

A second component of the CDC effort to build state and local capacities focuses on epidemiology: by providing funds for the hiring and training of epidemiology staff, providing local public health advisers and contacts from the Epidemic Intelligence Service trained to respond to bioterrorism incidents, developing enhanced communications and reporting mechanisms, and improving emergency notification procedures.

Events like World Trade Organization meetings in Seattle, Washington, and Washington, D.C., the Olympics in Atlanta, Georgia, and Salt Lake City, Utah, and national political conventions have provided test sites where improvements in both epidemiological and laboratory procedures could be explored. However, the huge workload generated by a few anthrax-loaded letters in October 2001 and the imitations and false alarms that they spawned pushed the current system to its limits and demonstrated the qualitative and quantitative needs for the rebuilding of the nation's public health system.

The CDC bioterrorism initiative has also built capacity within CDC itself by increased training of both laboratory and epidemiology staff and the development of communications technology like the Health Alert Network, which provides state and local health departments with essential computer hardware and software for interconnectivity, and expanded Internet access, which allows distance-based learning and access to the training institute at CDC. Another information technology initiative, the Epidemic Information Exchange program, provides epidemiologists with rapid access to information and advice from their peers. In the long term, a bioterrorism surveillance effort will be integrated into a National Electronic Disease Surveillance System covering a wide variety of activities and diseases.

Other activities under way at CDC include a national bioterrorism training plan for public health staff in state and local health departments; provision of guidance to health departments on epidemic control and how to forge useful relationships with emergency management, law enforcement, and the other components of government necessary for epidemic control; and a comprehensive examination of federal, state, and local quarantine authorities.

FEMA PROGRAMS

Among the many disaster preparedness programs and initiatives that FEMA makes available to individuals and communities are several that are especially relevant for the planning of responses to CBR terrorism and the present study of evaluation tools (Federal Emergency Management Agency, 1997a, 1999c).

Capability Assessment for Readiness

In partnership with the National Emergency Management Association (NEMA), FEMA developed a comprehensive self-assessment instrument to evaluate the operational readiness and capabilities of state emergency management programs (Federal Emergency Management Agency and National Emergency Management Association, 1997). The 1,801-element survey was administered to all 56 states and territories in 1997 with the goal of eventually using the results to develop a national emergency management standard. The survey covers 13 functional areas, from knowledge of applicable laws and authorities and hazard management to public education and information and finance and administration. An "all-hazards" document (Federal Emergency Management Agency, 1997b, 2000a), Capability Assessment for Readiness (CAR), asks respondents about plans and activities common to most disasters (e.g., hazard assessment, laws and authorities, communications and warning). It contains only a handful of CBR agent-specific items. CAR respondents are left to decide how to deal with local variations, but they are nevertheless asked to provide a readiness rating for each item (a five-point readiness scale ranging from fully capable to not capable is provided). In an effort to analyze the local capabilities more systematically, as well as to provide local officials with a useful means of self-assessment, FEMA, NEMA, and the International Association of Emergency Managers are creating a Local CAR that is undergoing pilot testing in selected counties.

Comprehensive Hazmat Emergency Response-Capability Assessment Program

The Comprehensive Hazmat Emergency Response-Capability Assessment Program (CHER-CAP) is an exercise-based program that assists local communities and tribal governments with obtaining a greater understanding of hazmat risks, identifying planning deficiencies, updating plans, training first responders, and stimulating and testing the system for strengths and needed improvements (Federal Emergency Management Agency, 2001b). CHER-CAP also assists jurisdictions in identifying ways in which hazmat prevention and mitigation measures can be implemented to reduce hazmat-related emergencies and protect the public.

CHER-CAP is conducted in phases spanning 4 to 6 months. Communities interested in undertaking CHER-CAP notify their state emergency management agency. The state then selects jurisdictions for participation. To qualify for selection, a jurisdiction must have, at a minimum:

- an active Local Emergency Planning Committee (LEPC) with an emergency response plan,
- a commitment from a local industry partner in the jurisdiction to participate in the program, and
- the commitment and involvement of a key first responder agency in the jurisdiction to take the lead for the community.

Most CHER-CAP initiatives eventually include fire and police departments, emergency medical services, public works agencies, health and environmental agencies, public officials, and hospitals, in addition to industry and the local emergency management office.

After the state selects the participants, the FEMA CHER-CAP coordinator and LEPC hold an initial meeting to discuss the scope of CHER-CAP and the general time frame that will be needed to conduct the program. If the community then commits to undertake the program, it begins by gathering such information as the LEPC plan, existing mutual-aid agreements, agency-specific standard operating procedures, existing data on hazardous substances in the community, documentation regarding training previously undertaken, and estimates of training needs.

After discussions about the existing plans and procedures, communities then implement any suggested modifications that they deem appropriate. Local and state agency officials, industry, and the FEMA coordinator identify available training programs on the basis of identified needs. Tabletop exercises also may be conducted before the full-scale exercise. The full-scale exercise scenario and staging considerations are then developed with LEPC and other participating entities as a part of the training so that agencies prepare to test and demonstrate their skills in the final no-fault, full-scale exercise.

The final phase of CHER-CAP, a full-scale hazmat exercise, is staged with live props, such as tanker trucks, railcars, or fixed facilities, simulated smoke and leaking liquid (dyed water), and simulated casualties. CHER-CAP exercises involve a mass-casualty scenario. As such, they also can be used to test a community's ability to respond to a terrorist incident during the first critical hours. The CHER-CAP exercise, which typically involves 100 to 300 participants, is tailored to the specific hazmat risks that the community confronts. The evaluation is based on the objective criteria in 16 functional areas outlined in FEMA's Hazmat Exercise Evaluation Supplement (Federal Emergency Management Agency, 2001a). These areas range from law enforcement, hazmat team, and emergency center operations to medical facility operations, population protection, and postexercise analysis. Peer evaluators observe the exercise and record their observations in a standardized format. Fire operations are observed by evaluators from other fire departments, police operations are observed by evaluators from other police departments, hospital operations are observed by evaluators from other hospitals, and so on. The exercise takes approximately 4 hours and is followed by a postexercise analysis. A final report based on the peer reviewers' reports is submitted to the participants after the exercise.

National Emergency Training Center

FEMA's National Emergency Training Center campus in Emmitsburg, Maryland, 75 miles north of Washington, D.C., is the home of two organizations offering short training courses relevant to emergency responses to the release of CBR agents. The National Fire Academy offers a wide variety of short courses at the Emmitsburg campus through a program of resident instruction and through a variety of off-campus programs. Any person with substantial involvement in fire prevention and control, emergency medical services, or fire-related emergency management activities is eligible to apply for National Fire Academy courses. Among a number of hazmat and emergency services courses are several CBR terrorism-related courses developed with funding from DOJ. These are described above in the section on DOJ programs.

The Emergency Management Institute (EMI) provides training in emergency management practices through a nationwide program of resident and nonresident instruction. Each year approximately 4,000 students attend courses while in residence at EMI, whereas 100,000 individuals participate in the nonresident program sponsored by EMI and conducted by state emergency management agencies. Additionally, tens of thousands of individuals use EMI distance-learning programs such as independent study courses and the Emergency Education Network in their home communities. Users can download different course materials that are intended to help senior local government officials prepare for and respond to terrorist incidents.

Courses of relevance for MMRS program cities include those on radiological monitors and operations during radiological incidents, exercise design and evaluation, and incidents with mass fatalities. Of special note are several courses aimed at local government officials responsible for planning responses to incidents of CBR terrorism. Under the general title Terrorism Consequence Management: Weapons of Mass Destruction Courses, a series of five facilitator-led courses is intended to help senior local government officials prepare for and improve their abilities to manage and respond to mass-casualty terrorism incidents involving the use of WMD. Each course has the same five objectives, and each uses a different scenario (terrorism involving nuclear, radiological, sarin, VX, or anthrax agents) to enable participants to accomplish them (Federal Emergency Management Agency, 2001c). There are 1-day and 3-day versions of each of the five courses. There are no student manuals, and the facilitator must tailor the course for the specific community. At the completion of the training, local government officials should be able to

- exercise greater leadership in preparing for and managing the response to mass-casualty terrorism incidents involving a WMD through a better understanding of their jurisdiction's response capabilities;
- analyze the appropriateness of the plans, policies, procedures, and other preparedness elements currently in place to respond to and recover from a mass-casualty terrorist incident;
- determine the adequacy of the level of training of jurisdictional disaster and emergency management staff;
- determine the adequacy of the jurisdiction's resources (e.g., personnel, material, and personal protective and other equipment resources) to respond to and recover from a mass-casualty incident; and

• identify the elements required to coordinate local, state, and federal government responses to terrorist incidents involving a WMD.

Material from three of these courses (Federal Emergency Management Agency, 2001d,e,f) has been incorporated into the committee's suggested evaluation activities (see Chapter 8 and Appendix F).

Radiological Emergency Preparedness

Following the 1979 Three Mile Island nuclear power plant malfunction in Pennsylvania, President Carter transferred the federal lead role in off-site radiological emergency planning and preparedness activities from the U.S. Nuclear Regulatory Commission to FEMA (the U.S. Nuclear Regulatory Commission retains responsibility for the oversight of safety at the actual sites of power plants and other licensees). FEMA established the Radiological Emergency Preparedness program to (1) ensure that the public health and the safety of the population living around commercial nuclear power plants would be adequately protected in case of a radiological incident at a nuclear power plant and (2) inform and educate the public about radiological emergency preparedness. The mission of the Radiological Emergency Preparedness program entails ensuring that adequate off-site emergency plans and preparedness programs are in place and can be implemented by state and local governments, a task which is carried out through the evaluation of scheduled biennial exercises (Federal Emergency Management Agency, 2000c, 2002c).

Chemical Stockpile Emergency Preparedness Program

For some years now, since the United States renounced the use of chemical weapons, certain kinds of chemical weapons have been stockpiled at eight U.S. Army installations in the continental United States while awaiting destruction. In the communities surrounding these installations, emergency plans and capabilities have been developed in recognition of the possibility of an emergency involving a chemical agent release. This effort, begun in 1988, is the Chemical Stockpile Emergency Preparedness Program (Federal Emergency Management Agency, 2001h).

The U.S. Army, as the custodian of the stockpiles, and FEMA, as the lead federal agency in preparing for and dealing with emergencies of all kinds, provide funds, guidance, resources, training, and other support. Each community makes emergency plans on the basis of its own unique needs and considerations. Planners consider the specific agents stored at the installation that is nearby, potential stockpile incidents that could put the off-post community at risk, various weather conditions, terrain, road systems, and other site-specific factors. Computers help community leaders evaluate and select the best protective measures for specific situations. Periodic exercises ensure that plans can be carried out rapidly and effectively.

4

Metropolitan Medical Response System Program Contracts

Any evaluation of the effectiveness of the Metropolitan Medical Response System (MMRS) program must involve examination not only of the capabilities of the participating cities but also the program's requirements. More simply, one needs to know not only how well the cities carried out the terms of their agreement with the U.S. Department of Health and Human Service's Office of Emergency Preparedness (OEP) but also whether those terms could reasonably be expected to result in enhanced capabilities for MMRS program cities. This chapter therefore describes those terms in some detail.

First, unlike many federal programs of assistance to state and local governments that provide funds by means of grants or cooperative agreements, OEP chose to use contracts as the mechanism for providing funds to participating MMRS program cities. The distinguishing characteristic of contracts is the level of detail provided in the "statement of work." Unlike grants, which often support desired processes and activities without specifying the expected product in any detail, contracts focus more closely on the products ("deliverables" in government jargon) and less closely on how the contractor is to produce them. This chapter examines the products that the MMRS program contracts require the cities to provide and touches briefly on the means by which OEP evaluates those products for compliance with the contract terms. Subsequent chapters focus on how to tell whether such compliance has resulted in a truly enhanced capability to respond to chemical, biological, and radiological (CBR) terrorism.

A second important and distinctive feature of the MMRS program is that the contracts bypass the state governments. Although cities are encouraged to involve surrounding jurisdictions and ensure that their plans are compatible with existing state emergency and disaster management plans, OEP has followed the lead of the U.S. Department of Defense (DOD), which was designated the lead federal agency by the Defense Against Weapons of Mass Destruction Act of 1996 (P.L. 104-201). The act, among other provisions, required DOD to provide civilian personnel of federal, state, and local agencies with training and advice on emergency responses to the use or threatened use of weapons of mass destruction (WMD). DOD decided to carry out that charge by providing training to the 120 cities with the largest core populations, which equates to all U.S. cities with populations greater than 144,000 in the 1990 census. The populations of those 120 cities represent about 22 percent of the U.S. population and are located in 38 states and the District of Columbia. OEP logically sought to leverage its MMRS program efforts by focusing on the jurisdictions slated to receive DOD training. See Appendix C for a list of the MMRS program cities by the first fiscal year of their contract with OEP.

FUNCTIONAL AREAS COVERED

The basic strategy of the MMRS program is to enhance local capabilities by organizing, equipping, and training local fire, rescue, medical, and other emergency management personnel to deal with the consequences of a terrorist attack with CBR agents. These personnel, usually a subset of emergency personnel that is tailored to each city, receive training on military chemical and biological agents; specialized protective, detection, diagnostic, decontamination, communications, and medical equipment; antidotes, antibiotics, and other pharmaceuticals and medical supplies; and enhanced emergency medical transport and emergency department capabilities. The program seeks to enhance capabilities in other areas as well, including threat assessment, public affairs, epidemiological investigation, expedient hazard reduction, mass-casualty care, mental health support, victim identification, and mortuary services. Perhaps the most important component of the program is the planning and organization that is required to identify and involve all the local, state, and federal offices and agencies with relevant resources, responsibilities, knowledge, and skills.

Despite some changes in the wording of the contracts and the number and nature of the deliverables since 1997, the core content of the MMRS program contracts covers the following activities:

1. detection and identification of the toxic agent or disease,
2. extraction of victims from contaminated areas,

3. decontamination of exposed persons (chemical or radiological incidents) and control of infection (biological incidents),
4. emergency treatment of victims,
5. triage and patient transport to definitive care,
6. definitive care,
7. mass immunization or prophylaxis,
8. mass fatality management, and
9. environmental surety (identifying residual health risk).

PRODUCTS DEMANDED

As noted earlier in the report, the original concept of a stand-alone Metropolitan Medical Strike Team (MMST), focused in large measure on augmenting existing hazardous material (hazmat) and emergency medical services in the event of an obvious multivictim attack involving a chemical weapon, has evolved into support for a wider-ranging system for responding to a variety of terrorism incidents. As a result, the products demanded of the contracting cities have changed since the program began in 1997. For example, all 1997 contracts were later amended (and additional funding was provided) to require a much more detailed plan for addressing biological terrorism incidents. Contractors were asked to plan responses for incidents of three different magnitudes: those with up to 100 victims, those with more than 100 but less than 10,000 victims, and those with more than 10,000 victims. Extensive guidance was provided in the statement of work, and 6 new deliverables were specified, in addition to the 10 required by the initial 12-month agreement.

The contracts awarded in fiscal years 1999, 2000, and 2001 are very similar to one another, although they differ in a number of respects from the fiscal year 1997 contracts (no new MMRS program contracts were awarded in fiscal year 1998). The 1997 cities' "bioterrorism supplement" was incorporated into the body of the contract in subsequent years, albeit with far less detail in the statement of work. Another change allows cities to build the capabilities of an MMST into their existing response organizations rather than create a stand-alone team. Smaller changes clarified OEP's intent in a number of places and provided cities with additional information about acceptable actions in others. No substantive requirements were added or deleted, and so, in the interests of brevity, only the provisions of the fiscal year 2000 MMRS program contract are presented here.

MMRS Program 2000 Contracts

Contracts awarded to the fiscal year 2000 MMRS program cities are

18 months in duration and call for the phased delivery of 12 products. The contracts also provide for an extension (Option 1) of 12 additional months to acquire the pharmaceuticals and equipment approved in the basic plan and any other actions necessary to make the MMRS operational. Exercising the option entails submission of monthly progress reports, a list of acquisitions, and a final addendum to the MMRS plan verifying demonstrated operational capability. The deliverables are numbered and printed in boldface, followed by the associated text from the contract statement of work. The comments of the Institute of Medicine Committee on Evaluation of the Metropolitan Medical Response Program are enclosed in brackets.

1. Meeting with Project Officer (within 2 weeks of contract award). Discuss the purpose of this contract and review key aspects of the accepted proposal.

2. The MMRS Development Plan (within 3 months of contract award) [the plan for developing a plan].

Outline the approach [who, what, when, how] to the creation of an enhanced ability to deal with a terrorist use of a weapon of mass destruction (WMD), and to identify how the public safety, public health, and health services sector responses to a terrorist incident will be coordinated. This MMRS Development Plan should detail the proposed leadership and membership of the development team and the philosophy underlying the proposed approach, along with a description of the geographic area that the plan will cover. The plan must also include a roster of the Steering Committee membership, representing the relevant organizations that will assist in the planning and development of the MMRS. Consideration should be given to the following Steering Committee membership: EMS [emergency medical services], EMS Project Medical Directors, public and private hospital representation, hospital ED [emergency department] representation from major receiving hospitals, local and state emergency management, Local Emergency Planning Committees, National Guard, local and state public health departments (infectious disease representation), mental health, the 911 system, poison control centers, Medical Examiner, local lab representation, police/FBI [Federal Bureau of Investigation] (including bomb squad), American Red Cross, and local federal agency representatives (i.e., DOD, VA, DOE, EPA, FEMA [U.S. Department of Defense, U.S. Department of Veterans Affairs, U.S. Department of Energy, the Environmental Protection Agency, and the Federal Emergency Management Agency]) where available.

3. Primary MMRS Plan (within 6 months of contract award).

Develop a Primary Metropolitan Medical Response System (MMRS) Plan for managing the human health consequences of a terrorist incident involving the use of weapons of mass destruction (WMD), i.e., a nuclear, radiological, biological and/or chemical device capable of creating mass casualties. The MMRS is considered to be an enhanced local capability for an existing system. The MMRS plan must interface with the state plan, and should be coordinated with other appropriate political jurisdictions (e.g., county government), with nearby/neighboring emergency response systems, and with nearby/neighboring MMRS systems (within approximately 25 miles of those with which mutual aid is anticipated to be used). This plan should identify and accommodate resident federal/state assets that may be useful for the city/metropolitan area response plan.

The MMRS should develop plans: for command and control, for notification and alert procedures, for management of public affairs, for provision of accurate and timely information, for centralized communication control, for control of transportation assets, for management/augmentation of medical personnel, for management of medical supplies and equipment, for emergency management of legal issues and credentialing, for emergency management of patient tracking/record keeping, for augmentation of epidemiological services and support, for laboratory support, for crowd control, protection of treatment facilities and personnel, for establishing a schedule for exercises, and for assigning responsibility for after-action reports and addressing report findings. Mental health services should be designed for the care of emergency workers, victims and their families as well as others in the community who need special assistance in coping with the consequences of this type of event. Plans for the proper examination, care and disposition of any humans who do not survive the attack should be included.

4. Component MMRS Plan for forward movement of patients utilizing the NDMS [National Disaster Medical System] (within 8 months of contract award).

To the extent that local resources are insufficient to provide the definitive health care required for all of those directly affected by the attack, develop a component of the MMRS Plan for forward movement of patients to other areas of the region or nation. An important consideration here is: who will make the decision to implement the forward movement of patients? This transportation and care would be provided by the National Disaster Medical System (this plan should be developed in coordination with the applicable Federal Coordinating Hospital).

5. Component MMRS Plan for responding to a chemical, radiological, nuclear, or explosive WMD event [NOT biological] **(within 9 months of contract award).**

Develop a component of the MMRS Plan for responding to and managing the health consequences of an incident resulting from the use of a chemical, radiological, nuclear, and explosive WMD. The MMRS should be able to detect and identify the weapon material or agent, extract the victims, administer the appropriate antidote, decontaminate victims, triage them and provide primary care prior to their transportation to a definitive medical care facility. The MMRS shall include plans for emergency medical transportation of the patients as well as emergency and inpatient services in hospitals that have the capacity and capability to provide the definitive medical care required, or to pre-designated off-site treatment facilities. Management of patients arriving at hospitals without prior field treatment/screening or decontamination should also be part of the MMRS. This plan shall also include procurement and provision of appropriate pharmaceuticals (sufficient to provide care for up to 1,000 victims), equipment, and supplies consistent with the mission and the MMRS. No pharmaceuticals or antidotes may be purchased until the list has been submitted to, and approved by, the Project Officer.

6. Component plan for MMST if it is a component of your MMRS (within 12 months of contract award).

If a clearly identifiable Metropolitan Medical Strike Team (MMST) is a component of your MMRS Plan, develop a component of the MMRS Plan for MMST capability that includes its mission statement, organization, membership, and concept of operations. Included in this operational plan shall be provisions for its activation, deployment, CBR agent identification, extraction of victims from the incident site, antidote administration, human decontamination, triage and primary care, and preparation of victims for transportation to definitive care facilities with sufficient supplies of appropriate antidotes to assure adequate treatment.

7. Component plan for managing the health consequences of a biological WMD (within 18 months of contract award).

Develop a component of the MMRS Plan to manage the health consequences of the release of a biological weapon of mass destruction. This plan should be integrated with existing or planned local and state health surveillance plans for bioterrorism and influenza pandemic planning. This portion of the plan should address five general areas.

(1) Early Recognition: The contractor should identify, describe, or develop early warning indicator(s) which will be used to alert local officials of a biological terrorist event, ensuring timely notification and activation of response plans. This plan should identify who will receive notification, and who will make the decision to further implement response plans.

(2) Mass Immunization/Prophylaxis: In this section, the contractor should highlight, develop, or augment existing plans for managing and implementing mass immunization/prophylaxis. In developing this plan, it should be assumed that the Federal government would assure the availability of vaccines and antibiotics within 24 hours of notification. Key components of this plan include a description of the decision making pro-

cess to initiate a mass immunization campaign, together with plans for identifying the affected population.

(3) Mass Patient Care: In this section, the contractor should develop or augment existing plans for providing care for a significant portion of the population. Key components of this plan include plans for rapid expansion of existing healthcare system capacity, and plans for taking care of people in excess of either existing or expanded capacity.

(4) Mass Fatality Management: In this section, the contractor should develop or augment existing plans for providing respectful care and disposition for a large percentage of the population. Key components of this plan are plans for augmenting existing morgue facilities and staff, and plans for decontamination/isolation procedures where appropriate.

(5) Environmental Surety: In this section, the contractor should describe or develop a plan for identifying environmental risk, need for decontamination or vector intervention, and a process for safe re-entry into a suspect area in consultation with local, state, and federal environmental agencies.

The size and robustness of any response to the use of a biological WMD will be determined by the specific biological agent. As a result, response planning should be considered at three (3) levels:

a. Incidents with up to one hundred (100) victims,
b. Incidents with one hundred (100) to ten thousand (10,000) victims,
c. Incidents with more than ten thousand (10,000) victims.

A detailed list of biological response planning considerations is included as an attachment. (This list is meant for your use as a planning tool only; it is not meant to be prescriptive in any way). A list of biological agents that should be considered is included as an appendix. [Those responsible for smallpox, anthrax, plague, botulism, tularemia, and hemorrhagic fever. The agent responsible for brucellosis was included in 1997 contracts, but those responsible for botulism and hemorrhagic fever were not.]

8. Component plan for local hospital healthcare system (within 18 months of contract award).

Develop a component of the MMRS Plan for the local hospital and healthcare system. Current JCAHO [Joint Commission on Accreditation of Healthcare Organizations] standards for emergency preparedness address an emergency preparedness management plan (EC.1.6), a security management plan (EC.1.4), hazardous materials and waste management plan (EC.1.5), and emergency preparedness drills (EC.2.9).

Ensure that this portion of the plan addresses the following eight general areas.

(1) Plans for notification of hospitals, clinics, HMOs [health maintenance organizations], etc., that an incident has occurred.

(2) Plans and procedures in place for hospitals, clinics, and HMOs to protect them from contamination from environmental or patient sources.

(3) Plans for providing triage and initiation of definitive care at local healthcare facilities.

(4) Plans for adequate security to support these activities.

(5) Availability of adequate personal protective equipment for hospital and clinic providers.

(6) Adequate pharmaceuticals and equipment (ventilators) are available locally, or that plans are in place to obtain them in a timely manner.

(7) Ability of medical staff to recognize and treat casualties caused by WMD agents.

(8) Treatment protocols are readily available.

9. MMRS Training Plan including training requirements and a follow-on Training Plan (within 18 months of contract award).

Develop a Training Plan for the MMRS that identifies training requirements for MMRS personnel, including all first responders, EMTs [emergency medical technicians], paramedics, vehicle drivers, emergency department and other hospital personnel who will be providing care to victims of a WMD incident. In the event that the DOD Domestic Preparedness training has been provided to the city, the contractor should indicate how the training received, including FEMA/DOJ training, will be integrated into meeting the initial training requirements as well as continuing education and other refresher training needs. For the training of hospital personnel, it is important to note that Presidential Decision Directive 62 (PDD 62) highlights the VA's role in the training of medical personnel in NDMS hospitals.

10. MMRS pharmaceutical and equipment plan that includes a maintenance plan and a procurement timetable for equipment and pharmaceuticals approved by the Project Officer (within 18 months of contract award).

Submit a list of pharmaceuticals consistent with the mission of the MMRS. Pharmaceuticals should be sufficient to provide care for at least 1,000 victims for a chemical incident, and for the affected population for the first 24 hours of response for a biological incident (it should be assumed that the Federal government would assure the availability of vaccines and antibiotics within 24 hours of notification). Equipment may include personal protective equipment, detection equipment and decontamination equipment (both field and hospital). A timetable for procurement of the above items and a plan for equipment maintenance and pharmaceutical storage should accompany this. A property officer responsible for all property received and purchased under this contract shall be identified. Equipment purchases under this contract must be harmonized with equipment received from DOD, DOJ, and FEMA programs. Only equipment and pharmaceuticals approved by the Project Officer shall be purchased under this contract.

11. Monthly progress reports and a final report 18 months after contract award.

These reports should describe successful endeavors and barriers encountered. Any barrier encountered should be accompanied with a plan to resolve the issue. Include all meeting minutes that relate to MMRS development.

12. Option 1 deliverables [if the city's MMRS is not operational upon submission of the final report] **are: a detailed list of equipment and pharmaceuticals acquisitions, continued monthly progress reports, and a final addendum to the primary MMRS plan certifying that the MMRS is operational.**

Carry out remaining actions that are required to assure that the MMRS is operational, including acquisition of pharmaceuticals and equipment as identified, planned and approved in deliverable #10. Continue to submit brief monthly progress reports and a final report at the end of the contract period. The final report must constitute an assessment of response capabilities (enhanced or created) that exist now as a result of the MMRS planning effort. The report shall identify actual equipment and pharmaceuticals procured and received under the contract. Identify additional assets/requirements that you will look to the Federal government to provide. These additional assets must be addressed in an addendum to the Primary MMRS Plan. The final report must include a statement that the MMRS has demonstrated operational capability. The final report shall be presented to the Project Officer no later than 12 months from the effective date of the option period.

CONTRACT DELIVERABLE EVALUATION INSTRUMENT

OEP staff uses the Contract Deliverable Evaluation Instrument to determine whether the contractor has met the terms of the contract, that is, has provided all the required deliverables and addressed all the elements of those deliverables specified in the contract. The contractor is encouraged to use the same instrument as a guide to action throughout the contract. Appendix D provides a copy of the checklist for the cities whose contracts began in fiscal year 2000. It served as the starting point and framework for the committee's analysis of potential preparedness indicators that is described in Chapter 6 and Appendix E.

5

Measurement and Data Collection in Evaluation

This chapter provides an overview of evaluation concepts and introduces some principles for their application to the Metropolitan Medical Response System (MMRS) program. Evaluation has been defined in numerous ways, but all of the definitions refer in some way to a systematic assessment to reach a judgment about value or worth (Scriven, 1991). The entity being evaluated can be a program, product, policy, or personnel. In the MMRS program context, the judgment about value might apply to

1. individual elements or components of an individual city's MMRS,
2. the capacity and overall performance of a city's MMRS,
3. the capacity and performance of the aggregate of city MMRS across the nation,
4. administration of the federal MMRS program or related agencies, and
5. federal- or state-level policies as they affect the adequate development of an MMRS.

Systematic assessment is a means to distinguish evaluation from subjective impressions or anecdotal evidence. Systematic assessment may be qualitative or quantitative in nature, but in all cases it is self-conscious about the need for validity and reliability in the assessment. *Validity* means (1) that independent assessors can agree on the relevance and appropriateness of criteria for judging value and on evidence that reflects those criteria and (2) that safeguards are in place to control potential bias in measurement, data collection, analysis, and the drawing of conclusions (Shadish et al., 2001). *Reliability* means that different assessors would reach similar conclusions on the basis of the evaluation methods used.

The context of the MMRS program presents some special challenges in terms of evaluation of the program. First, the MMRS program involves a web of planning activities, resources, intergovernmental agreements, and exercises at multiple levels of government. This web of activities is seen in Figure 5-1. Any one of a number of policy instruments, development activities, emergency capacity functions, and follow-up activities might be evaluated, or sets of them might be evaluated. Second, any MMRS itself represents an effort to coordinate multiple entities and activities that are independently funded and that receive their authority from other sources. Third, evaluation of the MMRS program is inferential, because even after September 11, 2001, incidents of domestic terrorism have occurred in only a few cities, and so the adequacies of most MMRSs have never been tested directly. Fourth, evaluation of the MMRS program is also inferential because, of necessity, assumptions must be made about how the component parts should work together.

EVALUATIONS OF VARIOUS TYPES

Evaluation can focus on a variety of entities and questions, such as the following:

- *Inputs.* Inputs are an individual city's resources, personnel, and political and logistic agreements committed on behalf of the MMRS.
- *Processes.* Also known as *implementation*, processes would include the variety of activities designed to achieve a specific level of capacity to detect an attack, to deal with the crisis phase, and to manage the aftermath. Such activities lead to the intermediate results required to achieve preparedness. These might include, for example, growth in decision makers' knowledge and experience with the variety of events in question, training programs under way in various units, designation and assumption of responsibilities, purchase of necessary equipment and supplies, and periodic testing of communications.
- *Outputs.* Because true terrorist attacks are, fortunately, still rare, an assessment of the ultimate outcome of the MMRS is not likely to be available for many cities. Instead, intermediate outcomes, referred to hereafter as outputs, are more feasible and are represented by progress of various elements of the system in response to exercises, false alarms, and nonterrorism events. Immediate outputs might include, for example, the number or percentage of personnel passing specialized tests on chemical or biological weapons.

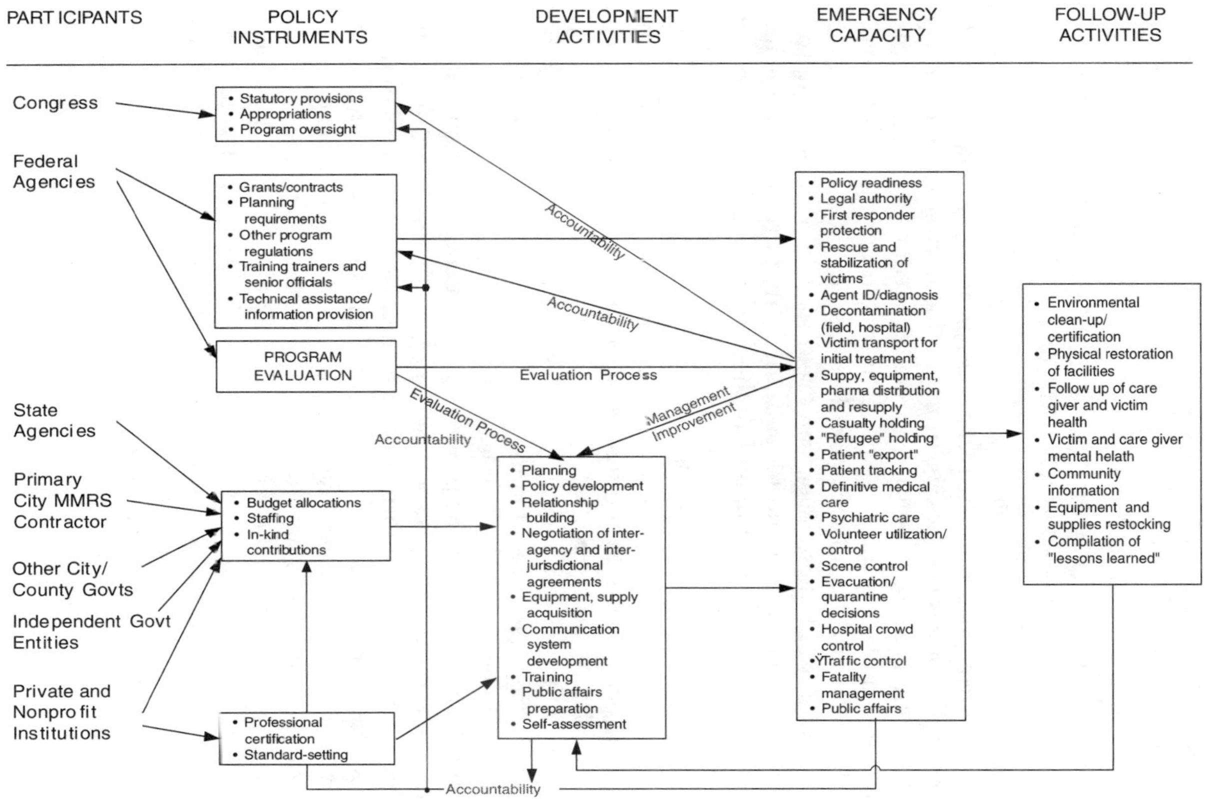

FIGURE 5-1 MMRS program participants, policy instruments, development activities, emergency capacity, and follow-up activities.

Other types of evaluations are sometimes distinguished, such as cost-benefit and cost-effectiveness analyses. These are less central to the questions posed by the Office of Emergency Preparedness (OEP) of the U.S. Department of Health and Human Services (DHHS) and so are not addressed here.

MANAGEMENT FUNCTIONS OF EVALUATIONS IN THE MMRS PROGRAM CONTEXT

The MMRS program provides a planning and coordination mechanism for cities' responses to chemical, biological, or radiological (CBR) terrorism that is otherwise lacking in the national capacity to deal with terrorist attacks. Because it aims to assist cities in coordinating a complex set of activities and capacities, the questions asked during evaluations of the MMRS program should focus on the federal, state, and city levels. Decision makers at all these levels can use these evaluations to improve the operation of the system and for accountability purposes. At the federal level, the primary aim is to ensure the maximum level of preparedness feasible in cities that vary greatly in terms of their resources and the levels of cooperation between participating agencies. At the city level, the need is to ensure a coordinated response among disparate agencies and units that are accountable to and funded by a wide array of federal, state, and local decision-making bodies.

Quite commonly, funding agencies, legislative overseers, and other stakeholders use program evaluation as a device to hold program managers or grantee agencies accountable. Evaluation results can help determine, for example, whether the program is producing expected substantive outputs, carrying out planned activities, and using grant funds for allowable purposes. This information can then be used to make future decisions about the program or an individual grantee. However, holding program managers or grantees accountable for their stewardship of a public mission or resources is not the sole purpose for which the results of evaluations can be used. Evaluation results can also be usefully applied to improve management of the program as a whole or of individual contracts or grants. Here the objective is to diagnose how well the program as a whole or individual grantees are performing with the objective of remedying shortcomings and identifying and replicating best practices. For a program that is likely to continue irrespective of current levels of performance because its substantive purpose is regarded as a critical public need, the management improvement function of program evaluations may well be as important as or more important than accountability.

Accountability Function

In the case of a specific program (e.g., the MMRS program), the key accountability relationship may extend from the federal agency or unit responsible for administering the program as a whole to higher-level department executives, the President and the federal Office of Management and Budget (OMB), and federal congressional authorizing and appropriations committees; more generally, it may extend to stakeholder groups and the public. Alternatively, the primary accountability relationship may extend from individual grantees back to the federal agency (see Figure 5-2).

The accountability function is often the prime motivation for evaluation requirements in federal grant programs. The information gathered during evaluations to assess accountability is useful in determining whether future funding commitments should be made in an agency's internal budget preparation process or in the congressional appropriations process, showing stakeholder groups that a problem is being effectively handled, or determining whether to reward a specific grantee with additional resources (or, possibly, not to renew or complete funding).

In each of these cases, the information generated during an evaluation is primarily used by external program overseers or stakeholders. The term often used for this is *summative evaluation* (Scriven, 1991). These re-

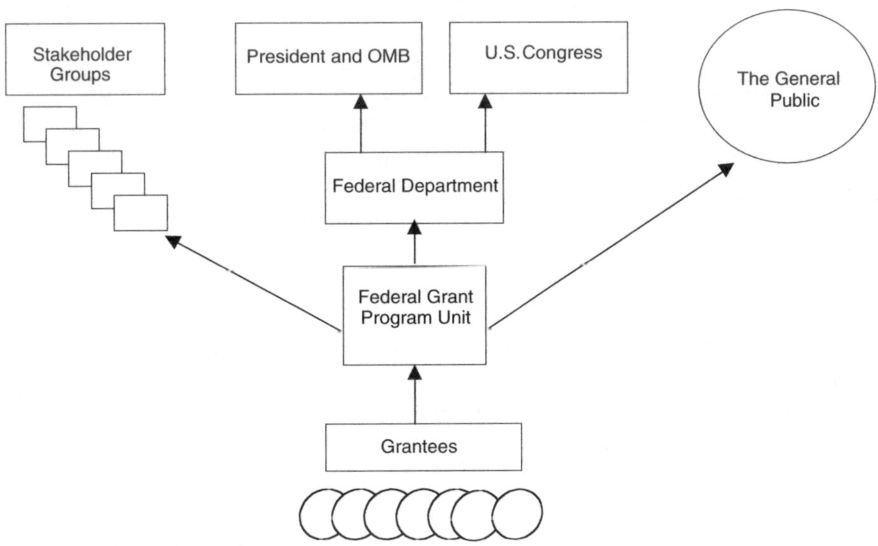

FIGURE 5-2 Accountability relationships for federal grantees and grant-making agencies.

cipients are rating or judging the adequacy of the program or the grantee's performance and deciding whether to act on the basis of this information. Although a grantee could benefit from a favorable rating (through an enhanced reputation or supplementary support), the evaluation performed for accountability purposes is not primarily oriented toward helping the program or the grantee. The program or the individual grantee is potentially at risk. Unfavorable judgments may bring negative consequences.

Management Improvement Function

Accountability is not the sole purpose of an evaluation. Instead, evaluations can be designed with the aim of helping the evaluated entity—whether it is the program as a whole or an individual grantee—assess its strengths and weaknesses and take appropriate future actions. This type of evaluation is termed a *formative evaluation* (Scriven, 1991). It can be closely related to technical assistance efforts (e.g., when OEP provides data to a city MMRS) and also to continuous quality improvement efforts (e.g., when a city MMRS makes use of locally collected data for local purposes).

The key characteristic of this approach is to emphasize feedback from the evaluators to those who have been evaluated—either individually or as part of a professional community that can share lessons and ideas to improve the overall performance of that community. When the evaluation reveals shortcomings, the follow-up step would be for the program or grantee or for outsiders to develop a course of action that would improve the program's capacity to at least satisfactory levels. When strengths are discovered, analysis can suggest whether there are lessons to be learned (either general lessons or lessons limited to certain contingencies) that might assist other grantees or similar entities. In that case, efforts can be made to use this information to work with less capable grantees or to disseminate information about best practices more widely.

Compatibility of Approach

Accountability and management improvement are not antagonistic conceptions of the purpose of evaluations. In principle, one could design procedures that would serve both functions. However, there are some definite tensions between these purposes:

- Managers in grantee organizations are more likely to feel wary of and are less likely to be cooperative with evaluations undertaken primarily for accountability purposes than with those aimed at management improvement.

• Evaluations aimed at management improvement are necessarily more customized, focusing on specific features of a particular environment, whereas accountability evaluations are likely to emphasize features standardized across jurisdictions.

• Limited resources may require the evaluating entity to set priorities among alternative purposes if implementation of a more wide-ranging evaluation is fiscally or administratively infeasible.

In what follows, the need to serve various evaluation audiences at the federal, state, and local levels will be termed "the layering problem," and the strategy used to inform these audiences through systematic data collection will be termed "the layering strategy." One feature of such a strategy might be to collect information that can be used by more than one audience. Some suggestions for the layering strategy will be offered in Chapter 9. However, the reality is that federal managers are likely to motivate most of the evaluations that occur and to push for the use of most of the data from those evaluations at other levels.

SUMMATIVE AND FORMATIVE USES OF VARIOUS EVALUATION TYPES

Many misconceptions arise in using the terms summative and formative evaluations for evaluation functions. In the case of the MMRS program, as with many programs, both formative and summative evaluations are ideally ongoing or are occurring on a cyclical basis. Evaluations can and do serve both formative and summative purposes at the same time. As noted previously, the same evaluation information can be used at both the federal (or state) and local levels (Leviton and Boruch, 1983). In addition, information from both formative and summative evaluations could be used in rhetorical or persuasive fashion, for example, to argue for additional funds or coordination at the federal level or to alert a key unit in the city's overall response plan that its personnel need improved training.

There is no hard-and-fast rule concerning the functions themselves. For example, federal decision makers often request information intending to make summative judgments, but they often use the information in a formative fashion to "tinker" with programs (Cronbach et al., 1980; Leviton, 1987; Leviton and Boruch, 1983). In the federal MMRS program context, OEP might indicate to a city that it had made satisfactory progress in building MMRS capacity, a summative judgment of worth, and then go on to indicate areas that still required improvement, a formative judgment.

A formative evaluation is sometimes equated with a process evaluation, and a summative evaluation is sometimes equated with an outcome or output evaluation. This conflates the function of an evaluation with the entity being evaluated. Processes and even inputs can be evaluated in a summative fashion, whereas outcomes are frequently used for formative purposes. Consider, for example, the following potential evaluations:

- OEP might indicate to a city that it had all of the requisite units and responsible parties in place, an evaluation of inputs and a summative judgment. At the aggregate level, OEP might report to the U.S. Congress the number of MMRS program cities that had these requisite inputs in place, a summative judgment. Yet, Congress might then request information about how to overcome barriers to getting these requisite inputs in place, a formative question.
- OEP might also indicate that an MMRS program city had not engaged in a satisfactory number of situational exercises or drills within the past year, an evaluation of process and a summative judgment. However, visitors to the site for the purposes of peer review might point out this obstacle and offer suggestions for overcoming it. For all MMRS program cities, OEP might report to DHHS or the Congress on the number of cities engaging in a satisfactory number of exercises, a summative statement, or it might report on typical barriers to achieving a satisfactory number of exercises, a formative statement.
- OEP or state- or city-level evaluators might determine that a component system in a city's MMRS does not meet the standard for speed of mobilization. This is a summative judgment about outputs. For all MMRS program cities, OEP might indicate the number of cities whose systems do not meet the standard, also a summative statement. However, peer reviewers working in the spirit of quality improvement might probe in-depth with cities not meeting the standard to determine barriers and to make suggestions on how failure to meet the standard can be overcome. This is a formative evaluation activity.

WHY AN ADEQUATE WRITTEN PLAN IS NOT SUFFICIENT ASSURANCE OF PREPAREDNESS

To date, OEP staff have used a checklist format to assess whether cities' plans for their MMRS included the component parts that would be necessary to achieve preparedness (see Appendix D). Assessment with the checklist has been followed by personal contact and observation in many cases, and this has permitted OEP staff to use their substantial experience in judging more directly whether a city's plans were adequate. Although this format has been an important starting point for evaluations of local systems, it has served primarily to ascertain whether local planners had included the variety of important inputs in their written plans.

Changing the format from a simple yes/no checklist to a graded instrument with potential answers ranging from "absent" to "exceptional" would help both OEP and contractor communities identify weaknesses to be shored up and strengths worth sharing with other communities. However, as municipal systems develop further and more contract experience is gained, OEP has recognized that the checklist alone is insufficient grounds for concluding that an MMRS program city is in fact prepared to cope with the consequences of an act of terrorism involving a CBR agent. The checklist is described below, followed by some reasons why it is not sufficient. The following section then examines a variety of alternative ways to measure the performance and outcomes of an MMRS.

1. A checklist format is insensitive to matters of degree. As such, it does not adequately reflect reality. It measures variables in a categorical, dichotomous fashion, assessing whether or not a system or function meets a standard or has adequate capacity. In reality, there are degrees of preparedness. Each community would cope with a terrorist attack to the best of its ability, and even if all standards were met, "success" would still be a matter of degree. Also, the MMRS program can set and encourage standards, but in the event of an attack, more can be learned from assessing the degree to which performance standards were achieved than from merely noting whether a standard was met.

2. A checklist does not permit recording of the information that can be used to improve an MMRS. Although the checklist indicates functions that are not available and that need to be addressed, it does not indicate the actions that a city should be taking to further increase its capabilities in specific areas.

3. The MMRS program cities must have the capacities to deal with a great variety of potential incidents. The sheer number of possible variations in terrorist incidents (the weapon used, the mode of delivery, the range of crisis capacities that are essential or that could be used, the targets of the terrorist attack, and relevant aspects of the urban situation) means that even though the preparations may be perfect for one incident, they may have limited applicability to another incident. The checklist format captures the range of capacities that might be needed only in the broadest way.

4. A checklist to assess a plan on paper is seldom an adequate reflection of local reality. In general, a small number of individuals write the existing plans. Even with the best will in the world, these individuals may not fully appreciate either the limitations or the actual crisis capacities possessed by other agencies that need to be part of the system. Local politics that undermines coordination may not be properly understood, or it may not be reflected in the plan.

5. A written plan does not present a test of operational conditions. Observations under several operational conditions are vital to achieving confidence in the eventual success of an MMRS: (a) a test of the plan under exercise conditions, (b) a test under a variety of real emergencies (both terrorist and nonterrorist in nature), and (c) a test under conditions in which the MMRS is confronted with unexpected conditions or when parts of the plan fail. Murphy's Law should be assumed, and the availability of backup plans for each component is desirable.

6. A checklist to assess a plan on paper is vulnerable to "corruption of indicators." It has long been understood in evaluations of health and social programs that when rewards and punishments result from people's apparent performance on an indicator, that indicator can sometimes change in ways that have no bearing on the actual outcomes of a governmental system (Blau, 1963; Campbell, 1988). This produces a lack of validity (increase in bias) in reporting to OEP from the field. In the context of the MMRS program, at least two possible forces can lead to a corruption of indicators. First, municipalities may believe that continued federal funding is contingent on features of their plan; through self-reporting, the writers of the proposal for a grant may make the situation appear better than it is in reality. Second, even in the absence of such contingencies, no city manager wants the public to believe that the city is not prepared for emergencies. The committee heard from congressional staff of glowing reports about the results of exercises in several cities; in actuality, the cities had failed rather badly to protect their populations from potential harm from a weapon of mass destruction.

7. Capacity or preparedness for each of the functions and components of the MMRS program is inferred; it cannot be directly observed because there have been very few actual terrorist incidents in the United States. Even if abundant examples of terrorist events were available, the "crisis capacity" itself could be inferred only from the responses of many different players at the federal, state, and local levels operating within complex systems and reacting to complex events.

However, OEP personnel already infer crisis capacity in ways beyond the scope of the checklist that they use. On the basis of their expert understanding of what is required to address a terrorist incident with CBR weapons, OEP officials can assess a variety of features of a city's MMRS plan beyond what is on paper. What is needed is a way of systematizing those judgments in the most cost-effective way and in terms of the level of accuracy or validity that is justified by the cost, the response burden (the time required to fill out paperwork, participate in a site visit, and undergo interviews) for local contractors, and use of the time of scarce federal personnel to assess the MMRS programs. A checklist format offers one of a range of potential ways to infer the degree of crisis capacity for various MMRS functions.

Two conclusions follow from this description of the existing instrument. First, MMRS capacity or preparedness is more usefully viewed as a complex policy goal than an absolute set of conditions that can be directly ascertained. In this respect, MMRS capacity or preparedness is like other big policy goals discussed in the United States, for example, policies related to access to medical care, privacy, and child health and well-being. No single indicator can assess it directly. Second, these big policy goals are best achieved through the use of multiple measurement strategies since any individual measurement strategy is inevitably flawed. In what follows, the advantages and disadvantages of some of these measurement strategies are described. Later chapters outline specific recommendations for measurement, data collection, and analysis.

EVALUATION MEASUREMENT FOR LOW-FREQUENCY, HIGH-STAKES EVENTS

As of this writing, a chemical, nuclear, or biological terrorist attack is a low-frequency, high-stakes event within the United States. As such, a terrorist attack presents challenges both to the maintenance of crisis capacity and to its improvement. In this respect, MMRS programs are similar to other systems and sets of skills with which it is a challenge to gain sufficient practice. For example, maintaining satisfactory skills for cardiopulmonary resuscitation requires refresher training (Baessler, 2000; Broomfield, 1996).

A central challenge in maintaining crisis capacity in a system that is preparing for a low-frequency event is the need for some form of ongoing feedback to address flaws in the component parts. Other systems have faced similar problems and have discovered various methods to assess preparedness for low-frequency events through the assessment of higher-frequency, more proximal events. For example, worker safety faces this challenge because, thankfully, serious injuries and fatalities do not happen very often in most workplaces in the United States. Therefore, those charged with preventing worker injuries have turned to proxies for accidents, such as monitoring behaviors and conditions on the job that pose a risk of injury. Dangerous behaviors and conditions are then addressed as soon as possible since it is well understood that learning is most effective when the behavior and its consequence are closely paired in time (Feldman, 1985; Komaki et al., 1978; Samways, 1983).

Two recommendations stand out as central:

1. For evaluation, as for feedback systems generally, measurement of the more frequent, more proximal indicators is a superior strategy. Therefore, the committee recommends the evaluation of outputs instead of outcomes. When outcomes are available, either in the wake of a true terrorist event or through proxy measures, they need thorough study as a basis for learning and improvement. They are not, however, the basis of an evaluation system.

2. Multiple kinds of indicators are likely to be necessary to give an adequate picture of the performances of an MMRS:

- Multiple indicators (whether they are outputs, processes, inputs, or proxy measures for actual incidents) permit quantification of the degree of preparedness or the capacities of the MMRS. Low-frequency events such as terrorist attacks offer measures that are not sensitive to real improvements because the level of measurement (disaster versus no disaster) provides far less information than a cumulative examination of proxy incidents over time.
- Proxy measures are important because substantial preparations may be made before an attack, but without a proxy measure their effectiveness will only become apparent in the aftermath of an attack, too late for corrective action.
- Indicators and proxy measures describe trends in performance over time. Thus, in keeping with the analogy of worker safety presented above, a supervisor tracking incidents of a worker's behavior that pose a danger to the worker or others can examine whether his or her approach to improving the safety of employees is working. In the same way, certain indicators recommended later in this report assess the speed with which component systems in a city are notified and involved in drills or situational exercises. If the trend is for the time to notification to be reduced, the city MMRS managers will have some confidence in the methods that they have chosen to improve responsiveness.
- Multiple kinds of indicators and liberal use of proxy measures are important because many and various types of terrorist incidents may occur. Success with dealing with one kind of attack, whether it is real or simulated, offers less assurance than one would like about whether other potential attacks would also be dealt with successfully. However, the use of many different kinds of incidents, events, and simulations as proxies for the variety of potential attacks that may occur offers more information on how these might be handled.

EVALUATION MEASUREMENT: PERFORMANCE MEASURES AND PROXIES

Provided that several assumptions are accepted, it is feasible to create two classes of measures for the MMRS program that are higher in frequency than actual incidents and that can be monitored more closely than an actual incident could. The two classes are proximal measures related to likely performance and proxies for actual incidents. In terms of performance, one of the theories underlying the MMRS program is the assumption that the component parts of the systems (e.g., the police, firefighting personnel, emergency medical services personnel, and epidemiologists) must perform adequately or the MMRS program will not perform adequately. Because the skills of the individuals who make up these component parts are periodically assessed, to the degree that their functions are relevant to the performance of the program in a terrorist incident, these assessments can partially represent the capacity of the MMRS.

The performances of the component parts of the MMRS program in response to various actual emergencies and incidents that bear some resemblance to what might occur in a terrorist attack could be assessed. Such incidents range from chemical spills (which would test the capacity to deal with hazardous materials), to medical system responsiveness to flu epidemics, to pranks (e.g., the release of pepper spray at a local mall or the mailing of letters falsely claiming to contain anthrax spores), to the turnaround time until the state epidemiology office is notified about the appearance of a cluster of suspicious cases of an infectious disease. Different components of the system are involved in many such incidents, and the assumption is that the performance of those components is relevant to what might happen in likely terrorist incidents. In this respect, after action reports about the performances of the various components of the system become crucial components for evaluation, especially for local system improvement.

Furthermore, such monitoring can also provide a means for establishing accountability of the MMRS to OEP, in line with the layering strategy for evaluation outlined above. Accountability can be achieved if OEP is satisfied that MMRS leadership is addressing problems identified either by OEP or by the local MMRS leadership. Alternatively, OEP may want to assess progress and establish a timetable to address a problem with one of the components of the MMRS. It is reasonable to hold the MMRS accountable for progress in addressing potential flaws. It is not reasonable to hold the MMRS accountable for all possible outcomes that might result from the endless variety of potential terrorist scenarios. In general, the use of these proximal measures and proxies will cost less than the use of some of the alternative strategies.

CRITERIA FOR SELECTION OF EVALUATION METHODS

A variety of methods might be of use in evaluating MMRS program cities. The choice of methods should depend on cost and feasibility, and the criteria presented below.

Resources and Skills in the National Program Office

The management improvement approach to evaluation may represent an additional responsibility for the national program office for which resources are lacking or inadequate. Conducting evaluations to spur management improvement, moreover, requires different skills for the national MMRS program staff than they may have available. Follow-up technical assistance depends on operational activities that are quite different from the contract writing and fiscal management tasks that characterize much of current program stewardship. Whether these skills are sufficiently developed in the existing national program office is an important question for which inadequate information to be able to provide an answer is available.

Developmental Phases

Because an MMRS is typically started from scratch in a particular jurisdiction and because its growth is then nurtured through a process that takes at least several years and it must then be sustained at a high level of readiness and competence for an indefinite period, each MMRS can be presumed to go through a series of developmental steps. There may be a high degree of similarity in the developmental phases encountered in each jurisdiction; alternatively, there may be idiosyncratic features in some or all jurisdictions that make it difficult to prescribe or foresee how development will proceed.

If evaluations are done across the board on a regular schedule, not all grantees will be at the same stage of development during any particular evaluation period. If evaluations are done for each grantee at specified intervals after a grant is given, the evaluation instrument and process can be designed to be sensitive to the developmental trajectory of the particular grantee.

The Federal Emergency Management Agency's National Urban Search and Rescue Team program may provide a model for the evaluation of an MMRS at different stages of development. The Urban Search and Rescue Team program uses a three-stage process designed with the idea of a progression of developmental phases. These stages are (1) a self-assessment in which a checklist of equipment and training steps is used, (2) a peer visit by recognized experts in the field who consider a set of operational guidelines, not just a checklist, and (3) a deployment exercise that helps determine whether the urban search and rescue team is ready for action.

Variations Among MMRS Program Cities' Resources

Evaluations of MMRS program cities must face the problem that some municipalities will never be able to afford the assets that protect other municipalities. In addition, municipalities often have special considerations: vulnerable targets that differ from those of other municipalities. For example, Washington, D.C., needs to anticipate likely attacks on numerous federal facilities and embassies, whereas Baton Rogue, Louisiana, has a variety of chemical plants that are vulnerable to attack.

One implication of these problems is that MMRS capacity and its assessment will need to be tailored, at least to some degree. Another implication of the variations in resources available to deal with a terrorist attack is that plans should have a hierarchy of methods to approach an incident; that is, backup plans should be available. These might be assessed at the time of application for the MMRS program contract, they might be suggested at the time of site visits, and they might be tested over time in much the same way that the more preferred plans are.

Timeliness of Feedback

The time between the gathering of evaluation information and the provision of feedback (whether it is formal and conclusive or informal and provisional) should be relatively short. Long delays mean that shortcomings may not be addressed as quickly as they could be or that the conclusions reached may be outmoded by further events or developments that have not been taken into account by the evaluation.

Communications Channels

Evaluations undertaken for management improvement purposes have less defined boundaries than evaluations undertaken for accountability purposes. One of the key side effects of such evaluations is therefore the establishment and densification of lines of communication from a grantee to other grantees and outside experts. These channels can be used for operational improvement purposes even after the evaluation is nominally complete.

To the extent that peer review is used (see Chapter 8), it should be noted that the learning is two way and is not limited to the jurisdiction being reviewed. Best-practice ideas may emerge and may deserve to be disseminated. The national meetings of MMRS officials could be incorporated in some fashion into the process of communicating insights from the evaluation process.

Measurement Characteristics

Most evaluations are a combination of qualitative and quantitative approaches, each of which brings strengths and weaknesses. Qualitative studies provide greater depth of understanding about a small number of cases or subjects, often identify new variables for study or new relationships among variables, but that understanding may not generalize beyond the few cases studied. Quantitative measures typically provide greater breadth of understanding and, depending on the research design, may allow for strong inferences about causation, but the depth of knowledge will be limited (Cronbach, 1982; Francisco et al., 2001). Both approaches must deal with the issues of reliability (Will the measures yield the same result in the hands of different evaluators?) and validity (Do the measures provide an accurate picture of reality, or make accurate predictions about future events?). The former can generally be assessed by comparing measurements of a small sample of cases by two or more evaluators, and this should be possible for any MMRS evaluation tools as well. Validity testing on the other hand relies on comparison of a condition or event predicted by the measurement instrument to an actual condition or event. In the case of MMRS preparedness, the actual event would be an effective response to a large-scale CBR terrorism incident, so validation of any preparedness measurement would depend on the occurrence of a large number of such incidents. In practice, the most important measurement characteristic may be response cost, the money, time, and energy required of the organizations being evaluated, for without the enthusiasm, or at least the willing cooperation of those organizations the evaluation is liable to be meaningless.

6

Preparedness Indicators

The Metropolitan Medical Response System (MMRS) program context presents some special challenges for evaluation. First, there is much to be learned from analysis of the local, state, and federal responses to the terrorist attacks on the World Trade Center and the Pentagon in September 2001; but the committee believes that chemical, biological, or radiological (CBR) terrorism incidents of the scale envisioned by the Office of Emergency Preparedness (OEP) of the U.S. Department of Health and Human Services are unlikely to occur on a regular basis. As a result, any evaluation of a response system will have to be indirect, in that it will have to measure the intermediate consequences of the MMRS program rather than the ultimate goal, which is to save lives and minimize morbidity from a terrorism incident.

Second, every city's MMRS encompasses a web of planning activities, resources, intergovernmental agreements, and exercises at multiple levels of government. This web of activities was illustrated in Figure 5-1 in Chapter 5. The many activities in the box beneath "Emergency Capacity" represent only some of the capabilities required for an effective response to CBR terrorism events. Producing those capabilities is the concern of a wide variety of governmental and private-sector institutions through an equally wide variety of mechanisms, including the MMRS program. The MMRS program itself represents an effort to coordinate multiple entities and activities that are independently funded and that receive the authority for their activities from other sources. This complexity means that isolation and quantification of OEP's role in creating readiness for a CBR terrorism incident will be nearly impossible, regardless of how well one might measure readiness in any given city. It also suggests that caution is called for in making changes in any part of the web of activities, for they may have unintended consequences far from the locus of change.

Third, although many of the pieces of a response plan may be thoroughly evaluated, evaluation of response capacity as a whole will, by necessity, be inferential; that is, assumptions must be made about how the component parts should work together.

Fourth, the wide variations in the resources and vulnerabilities of the MMRS program municipalities may preclude use of a single yardstick or measure that places all the MMRS cities along a single scale of readiness. As noted in the previous chapter, Washington, D.C., must anticipate attacks on numerous federal facilities and embassies, whereas Baton Rouge, Louisiana, has a variety of chemical plants that are vulnerable to attack. Some cities operate their own emergency medical services; others depend on private, county, or state assets. OEP has dealt with this variation by not attempting to impose a single model or acceptable plan on all its MMRS program cities, instead opting to encourage cities to build their own plans in conjunction with the available structures, resources, and vulnerabilities. This flexible approach results in a substantial reduction in the ability to impose universal performance measures and standards and a corresponding difficulty in devising fair and comparable evaluation tools.

Finally, the committee has been persuaded by both the first five observations and the written and oral explications of OEP that it should approach its tasks with a strong bias toward a formative rather than a summative evaluation. That is, the committee takes as a given that the primary goal of the proposed evaluation is constructive feedback both to OEP staff and to the MMRS program cities.

EXISTING STANDARDS

Many of the personnel, professions, organizations, and jobs referred to in the plans of MMRS program cities are governed by existing standards; some of these are legally mandated (Occupational Safety and Health Administration [OSHA] regulations), and others are voluntary. The following is a partial list of potentially relevant standards that the committee examined:

Joint Commission for Accreditation of Healthcare Organizations (JCAHCO)
- Standard EC.1.4—Emergency preparedness management plan
- Standard EC.2.9.1—Emergency preparedness drills
- Standard EC.1.4 (1997)—Security management plan
- Standard EC.1.5 (1997)—Hazardous materials and waste management plan

Commission on Accreditation of Ambulance Services Standards
Organization (includes disaster plan, yearly disaster simulations)
Management
Community relations and public affairs
Human resources
Clinical services
Safety
Equipment and facilities
Communications

National Public Health Performance Standards (Centers for Disease Control and Prevention [CDC])

National Fire Protection Association Standards
NFPA 471—Recommended Practice for Responding to Hazardous Materials Incidents
NFPA 472—Standard for Professional Competence of Responders to Hazardous Materials Incidents
NFPA 473—Standard for Competencies for EMS Personnel Responding to Hazardous Materials Incidents
NFPA 1600—Standard on Disaster/Emergency Management and Business Continuity Programs

OSHA Standard 29 C.F.R. § 1910.120)—Hazardous waste operations and emergency response

Nuclear Regulatory Agency and Federal Emergency Management Agency (FEMA) Criteria for Preparation and Evaluation of Radiological Emergency Response Plans and Preparedness in Support of Nuclear Power Plants (NUREG–0654/FEMA–REP–1)

U.S. Department of Transportation, National Highway Transportation Safety Agency, Emergency Medical Services, National Standard Curriculums

American College of Emergency Physicians Task Force Recommendations on Objectives, Content, and Competencies for Training of Emergency Medical Technicians, Emergency Physicians, and Emergency Nurses on Caring for Casualties of NBC (Nuclear, Biological, and Chemical) Incidents

With only a few exceptions, the committee deemed these standards to be of limited utility in assessing the preparedness of local communities for coping with a CBR terrorism incident. Although the National Emergency Management Association is in the process of developing an accreditation program (DeMers, 2001; National Emergency Management Association, 2001) that may ultimately serve as a means of evaluating most of the non-CBR agent-specific facets of an MMRS, most of the standards listed above are qualitative in nature and are "enforced" only by well-publicized and infrequent inspections. Most of them also focus on the adequacy of written plans, like the OEP checklist in Appendix D. None explicitly addresses CBR terrorism or an emergency of the scale described in the MMRS program contract, and attempts to apply these standards to such scenarios in the past have often proved counterproductive (e.g., misinterpretation of OSHA hazardous waste operations standards has led to expectations that hospital emergency department personnel should have Level A chemical protective suits). Furthermore, each standard applies to only one element, discipline, or agency involved in an MMRS.

It is difficult to envision a successful MMRS in which any of the constituent elements fails to meet its own narrow standards, but it is also true that a collection of individually competent elements does not guarantee a successful system. Each of the standards listed above was nevertheless examined for elements that could be incorporated into an MMRS-specific evaluation, and a number of those have been incorporated into the matrix of preparedness indicators provided in Appendix E.

EXISTING ASSESSMENT TOOLS

The committee examined the following assessment tools for possible application in whole or in part to the task of evaluating preparedness for CBR terrorism events:

Capability Assessment for Readiness (CAR)

—FEMA self-assessment instrument to evaluate state emergency management

—An 1,801-element survey administered to all states and territories in 1997

—"All-hazards" document with only a handful of items related to chemical and biological weapons

Local Capability Assessment for Readiness

—FEMA's smaller, local community version of CAR

—Currently undergoing pilot testing in selected counties

Hazardous Materials Exercise Evaluation Supplement

—Instructions and checklist for peer reviewers in FEMA's Comprehensive HAZMAT Emergency Response-Capability Assessment Program

—Sixteen elements, each with 10 to 50 "points of review"

—Yes-or-no responses and the time that the specific action was observed

Epidemiologic Capacity Assessment Guide

—Step 2 of a three-step process (Step 1 is document collection, and Step 3 is site visit) designed by the Council of State and Territorial Epidemiologists

—Self-assessment questionnaire

—Short answers or essays and data on speed of investigation from recent cases

—Suggestions for interviews of key personnel

State Domestic Preparedness Equipment Program Assessment and Strategy Development Tool Kit

—Instruments developed by the U.S. Department of Justice (DOJ), the Federal Bureau of Investigation, and CDC to evaluate vulnerability, threat, and public health system performance combined with assessments of required and current capabilities in the realms of fire services, hazmat services, emergency medical services, law enforcement, public works, public health, and emergency management

—A 100-page "Tool Kit" provided for use by the state and local personnel assigned to fill out the forms, but it could be the basis of peer interviews

—State assessment designed to be a compilation of local assessments, so it is really a local instrument

Public Health Assessment Instrument for Public Health Emergency Preparedness (CDC)

—Ten essential public health services amplified specifically for preparedness for CBR terrorism events

—Nineteen "indicators," each with multiple subparts requiring mostly yes-or-no answers

—Part of DOJ state assessment instrument

Assessment of Community Linkages in Response to a Bioterrorism Event

—Draft (Spring 2001) product of JCAHCO and SAIC, Inc., for the Agency for Healthcare Research and Quality

—Forty-item questionnaire for hospitals (yes-or-no and short answers)

Chemical and Bioterrorism Preparedness Checklist
—American Hospital Association 8-page self-analysis

Mass Casualty Disaster Plan Checklist: A Template for Healthcare Facilities
—A list of 135 items from the Association of Professionals in Infection Control and Epidemiology and the Center for the Study of Bioterrorism and Emerging Infections

Each of these instruments seeks information about elements of disaster preparedness that are directly relevant to CBR terrorism preparedness. All are written self-reports, and either of the two most comprehensive assessments, done properly, would take several people many hours or even several days to complete. In addition, the committee believes that self-reports are vulnerable to "corruption of indicators." It has long been understood in evaluations of health and social programs that when rewards and punishments result from people's performance on an indicator, that indicator can sometimes change in ways that have no bearing on the actual outcomes of the governmental program. In the context of the MMRS program, at least two possible forces can lead to corruption of indicators. First, to the extent that municipalities may believe that continued federal funding is contingent on contract compliance, self-reports may make the situation appear to be better than it really is. Second, and alternatively, if local officials believe that further funding is dependent on need, self-reporting may actually lead to an underestimation of preparedness. Like the existing standards described in the previous section, most of these instruments also focus on the adequacy of written plans, like the OEP checklist in Appendix D. In sum, the committee views them as providing too little additional assurance for the substantial effort involved.

The committee also sought information on how other countries assess their capabilities to respond to a terrorist attack with a CBR agent. The United Kingdom (UK) and Israel have faced terrorism for several decades, although conventional explosives have been the weapon employed in almost all cases, and no single incident has been of the magnitude envisioned by the MMRS program planners. Both of those countries' armed forces have active research and development programs in the chemical and biological defense realms and equip their troops very similarly to U.S. Forces. A recent paper by Sharp (2002) on counterterrorism preparation in UK cities noted that a free society cannot reveal all to its citizens, but implied that there is little evidence to back up the British government's assertion that it is both informed and prepared. The UK national medical system would presumably make the preparation task easier than it is in the United States, but the IOM Committee staff was unable to locate a description of an assessment program or procedure comparable to that being asked of the Committee.

Israeli measures to protect its citizenry from possible attack with chemical or biological weapons during the Persian Gulf war of 1991 are well-known. Danon and Shemer (1994) provide a large collection of papers on Israeli medical lessons from the Gulf war. Every person in Israel, for example, has a personal protection kit containing a gas mask, decontamination powder, and an autoinjector of atropine. In times of national strife all Israeli health services are coordinated through a Supreme Hospitalization authority and civilian and military patients become one pool. As a result civilian hospitals are closely involved in planning for the care of chemical and biological casualties. In fact all Israeli hospitals are expected to be able to manage a sudden influx of patients, in a mass casualty incident, of 20 percent of the number of the hospital's beds (Personal communication, Y. Waisman, Director, Unit of Emergency Medicine, Schneider Children's Medical Center of Israel, Petah-Tiqva, to F. Henretig, March 1, 2001). Their plans also assume that half of the patients would be moderately to critically ill and that 20 percent would be pediatric victims. Chemical warfare drills involving both emergency medical services and hospitals are conducted every 36 months, mass casualty drills every 18 months, and simulations with senior hospital and military staff every 12 months. An innovation the IOM Committee finds attractive is the use of "smart simulated casualties" in these drills—military physicians and recent graduates of an Advanced Trauma Life support course (Gofrit et al., 1997). Unpublished and undated briefing slides of Smuel Reznikovich made available to the IOM Commitee by K. Tonat, Office of Emergency Preparedness, reveal that Israeli hospitals are periodically evaluated for readiness on a 110 point scale. Evaluation covers 16 subjects, including personnel, training, logistics, medical equipment, blood bank and medications, and "chemical warfare deployment," but attempts to obtain further details were unsuccessful.

PERFORMANCE MEASURES VERSUS PREPAREDNESS INDICATORS

The MMRS contract deliverables are all written plans, and although written plans are certainly necessary elements of preparedness, they are in most cases only the beginning of a continuing process. Some elements of these plans can be carried out only during or after an actual incident or a very realistic exercise, but many require advance preparations, such as the purchase of equipment, hiring or training of personnel, or even changes in the way in which everyday business is conducted (for example, citywide electronic surveillance of emergency department visits or 911 calls). Even though these advance preparations and their documentation are actions and are necessary for preparedness, they are not the same sort of performances that might be assessed in an actual mass-casualty event (whether it involves CBR terrorism or not) or a drill or field exercise. Measures related to advance preparations are generally easier and cheaper to access, however, and can provide a measure of effective response capability or potential (although, in the absence of an act of mass-casualty-producing CBR terrorism, there are no data that can validate the relationship between the selected indicators and actual performance). The committee therefore prefers the more inclusive term "preparedness indicators" to "performance measures."

The committee's recommended preparedness indicators are presented in Appendix E as a series of tables. A separate table is provided for each of the substantive deliverables of the MMRS program's fiscal year (FY) 2000 contract (omitted are preparedness indicators for three deliverables that call for a meeting with the project officer, monthly progress reports, and a final report, respectively). In each table in Appendix E the far left column, labeled "Plan Elements," lists the required elements of the deliverable, numbered in accord with the checklist supplied to FY 2000 MMRS program cities by OEP under the title "2000 MMRS Contract Deliverable Evaluation Instrument," a copy of which is provided as Appendix D

The remaining three columns of the tables present the committee's suggested preparedness indicators for each plan element. These fall into three categories: inputs, processes, and outputs.

Inputs are the constituent parts called for, implicitly or explicitly, by a given deliverable. An adequate plan itself would contain at least one input for nearly every deliverable, assuming that the required plans would have been completed at the point that the assessment is being undertaken. Other inputs could be designated personnel; standard operating procedures; equipment and supplies; or schedules of planned meetings, training, and other future activities.

Processes are evidence of actions taken to support or implement the plan. Evidence that such actions had been taken or are under way might include minutes of meetings, copies of agreements that had been prepared, evidence that training sessions had been conducted, or the numbers or percentages of personnel trained to use CBR detection equipment.

Outputs are indicators of effective capabilities developed through the actions included under processes, that is, indicators of the effectiveness of actions taken to support or implement the MMRS program plan. They would include preparations that have been completed, for example, establishment of a stockpile of antidotes and antibiotics appropriate for the agents that pose the greatest threat, with evidence of adequate maintenance and deployment procedures. Another output would be demonstration of critical knowledge, skills, and abilities in tabletop exercises, full-scale drills, or surrogate incidents (deliberate scares and false alarms, unintentional chemical releases, naturally occurring epidemics, or isolated cases of rare diseases). Outputs may be evaluated through expert judgment by peer reviewers of answers to written questions or on-site probes. An important advantage of outputs is that they reflect intangibles not easily captured by the input and process indicators suggested by the committee. For example, a strong MMRS requires a champion with the desire and commitment to continually advocate for the project; individuals who are willing to cooperate; a change in attitude by organizational leadership that will adopt an interorganizational and systemic approach to the MMRS; and leaders from local, state, federal, and private agencies with trust and sensitivity to each other's missions, goals, strengths, and weaknesses.

The best evidence for preparedness will always be outputs, which are the end products of processes undertaken with inputs. A variety of circumstances, including the timing of the assessment, may make collection of output data impossible or impractical. In this circumstance evidence for preparedness might be sought among inputs and processes. All three types of indicators are, however, merely surrogate or proxy measures of MMRS effectiveness that are based on the judgment of knowledgeable students of the field but that have never been truly validated (and that cannot be, short of an actual mass-casualty CBR terrorism incident).

The tables in Appendix E present many preparedness indicators, in part because of the committee's decision to derive indicators for each of the items on OEP's checklist of elements required in the plan. In fact, no practical evaluation program could or should use all the indicators listed. Use of the output-based indicators, presented in the far right column of each table in Appendix E, provides the best means of assessing readiness, and whenever possible, these indicators should be used in preference to process- or input-based indicators. The importance of the output-based indicators, especially those obtained from exercises or careful evaluations of real disasters, cannot be overemphasized. Similarly, process-based indicators should take preference over input-based indicators. In addition, it should be clear that every element of the plan need not be given equal weight in the evaluation of preparedness. Indeed, it may not be necessary to include every element in even a very comprehensive evaluation. This selection and prioritization process is addressed in Chapter 8, as is determination of the most effective and efficient means of collecting the desired information and specifying some minimum standards for preparedness wherever possible.

7

Feedback to Office of Emergency Preparedness on Program Management

Although the focus of the work of the Institute of Medicine's (IOM's) Committee on the Evaluation of the Metropolitan Medical Response System Program was the preparedness of the communities around the United States that have developed or that are developing a Metropolitan Medical Response System (MMRS), a second part of the charge to the committee (see Chapter 1) concerns the performance of the U.S. Department of Health and Human Services' (DHHS's) Office of Emergency Preparedness (OEP) staff themselves in their administration of the program. The committee was asked how OEP can determine, at the program level (i.e., at the national level), whether the strategies, resources, mechanisms, technical assistance, and monitoring processes provided to the MMRS development process are effective.

The question of effectiveness cannot be fully answered independently of some measure of the preparedness of the MMRS program communities, a task undertaken in subsequent chapters. It cannot be overemphasized, however, that whatever the state of local preparedness, many programs and initiatives—those of the federal, state, and local governments and of the private sector—as well as preexisting conditions in each jurisdiction contribute to preparedness. It is therefore impossible, even for the MMRS program communities themselves, to fully disentangle the causal effects of the MMRS program relative to the effects of these other influences. It is nevertheless possible to make some judgments about OEP's administration of the program by asking its contractors, that is, the MMRS program communities, about the extent to which they used OEP technical assistance and resources in fulfilling the terms of their contracts, their perceptions of the value of that assistance and those resources, and how much fulfilling the terms of the contract improved community preparedness. A subsequent section of this chapter provides a suggested survey for administration to the OEP's primary point of contact in each MMRS program community.

That said, the committee believes that some independent analysis by the committee of the performance objectives identified in the MMRS program contract is both justified and desirable. Are they the right ones? Should there be more? That is, are the actions demanded of the MMRS program communities by their contracts with OEP necessary and sufficient for preparedness? Although these are questions for which input from the communities themselves would again be helpful and which cannot be fully answered before a full evaluation of local preparedness that presumably will follow publication of this committee's report, the committee nevertheless believes that several modifications and additions to the contract objectives ("deliverables") are very likely to enhance a community's response to an event involving a chemical, biological, or radiological (CBR) weapon.

OEP staff, the regional Public Health Service project officers, and the MMRS program contractors have identified two objectives as being especially important: Deliverable 2, the MMRS Development Plan, and Deliverable 8, Component Plan for Local Hospital and Healthcare System.

The required elements of Deliverable 2, the MMRS Development Plan, include specifying the proposed leadership and membership of a development team and the roster of a steering committee that will assist in planning and developing the MMRS. The contract suggests a number of organizations and agencies that should be considered, but variations among communities probably ensure that no list of suggested members will be appropriate for all communities. More importantly, the IOM committee has repeatedly heard that the real value of assembling a steering committee lies in the personal relationships established in the course of preparing the plan. Yet, nowhere in the guidance to the contractor on this deliverable is that stated explicitly. Also missing from the required elements of this deliverable is a preliminary assessment of the planning environment, that is, the community's strengths and weaknesses, opportunities and threats particular to that community, and any barriers and resources that might be unique to the community. A plan to enhance local capabilities should begin by identifying those capabilities in most need of enhancement. This should be a multidisciplinary effort offered by multiple voices in the community (e.g., police and fire departments, emergency medical services, public health agencies, and hospitals), with participation attested to by the signatures of all parties. The committee recognizes that this proposed addition to the list of deliverables comes too late for the 122 cities already under contract, but it believes that it would be the most logical start to any OEP initiative to provide follow-on support to sustain their readiness.

Deliverable 8, Component Plan for Local Hospital and Healthcare System, recognizes no distinction between public and private health care facilities, although it is clear from experience that some MMRS program contractors have had great difficulty involving private hospitals and clinics (see also U.S. General Accounting Office, 2001b). The contracts' guidance on this deliverable should include or refer the contractor to some strategies, mechanisms, or incentives for ensuring the involvement of private hospitals and clinics that have proved successful in other cities. In addition, the committee has identified two important elements of coping with a mass-casualty event that are not addressed in the objective: staff callback procedures and replenishment of medical and ancillary (food, laundry, housekeeping, etc.) supplies and services.

The committee also identified several other essential activities or MMRS functions that are not addressed at all in the current contracts:

- receipt and distribution of materials from the National Pharmaceutical Stockpile;
- evacuee care (shelter for healthy people fleeing an area of real or perceived contamination);
- volunteer utilization and management;
- traffic control at the scene of an event, at health care facilities, and in the community as a whole;
- evidence development, collection, and protection;
- decisions and procedures related to evacuation and disease containment;
- postevent follow-up of the health of responders and caregivers; and
- a plan for postevent amelioration of anxiety and feelings of vulnerability among the community at large.

It might be argued that several of these functions are not medical in nature and therefore do not fall within the scope of DHHS's MMRS program. However, all of these functions are essential to the ability of medical personnel to perform their jobs, even if, as seems likely, public safety personnel carry out the required actions. A realistic plan should therefore address these areas.

OEP HELP TO MMRS PROGRAM CONTRACTORS

OEP provides guidance and assistance to its contractor cities through a variety of mechanisms that extend well beyond simple specification of a series of performance objectives. These include the following:

- A detailed list of "planning considerations" for a bioterrorism plan. A collection of more than 130 issues in need of attention in any plan for coping with bioterrorism was appended to the 1999 modification to the fiscal year 1997 MMRS program contracts and all subsequent contracts.
- Regional project officer for consultation. Each of the 10 Public Health Service regions is assigned one to three regional emergency coordinators who also serve as the OEP project officers for the MMRS program cities within their regions. Many hold regular meetings with key personnel from their MMRS program cities, individually and as a group, for the exchange of information and advice.
- Yearly meeting of representatives from all MMRS program cities. In October 2000, OEP gathered representatives from all MMRS program cities for a development conference, intended to promote the exchange of ideas on how to address persistent problems in the planning process. This meeting will become an annual event, to be held 6 months after the annual meeting of the National Disaster Medical System, another OEP-sponsored event that includes a series of sessions devoted to MMRS program issues.
- List of contacts for all MMRS program cities. Distributed at the annual development conference, the list facilitates the sharing of information and solutions with other MMRS program cities.
- Public website with background materials, documents on terrorism, and links to other sources. The URL is http://www.mmrs.hhs.gov/Index.cfm.
- Secure website for key MMRS program personnel. A password is required for access to this site, which contains information of potential value to would-be terrorists. Access is restricted to a maximum of 15 designated individuals in each MMRS program city.
- Sample or model of a monthly report.
- Library of completed plans.
- OEP-funded research on common problem areas. Grants have been provided to a variety of institutions, including some cities that received MMRS program contracts in 1997, to devise and evaluate approaches to, for example, mass decontamination in cold weather, hospital decontamination systems, distribution of bulk drugs from the National Pharmaceutical Stockpile, electronic emergency department surveillance, and sustainment of preparedness after completion of the MMRS program contract. More recent contractors will presumably have access to the results of these studies.
- Checklist for self-evaluation of contract compliance. OEP staff use

a checklist, the Contract Deliverable Evaluation Instrument, to determine whether the contractor has met the terms of the contract, that is, has provided all the required deliverables and addressed all the elements of those deliverables specified in the contract. The contractor is encouraged to use the same instrument as a guide to action throughout the contract. Appendix D is a copy of the checklist for the cities awarded contracts in fiscal year 2000.

All of these efforts at helping MMRS program cities meet the terms of their contracts impress the committee as being potentially valuable, but the utility of this management assistance for both contract completion and effective preparation for CBR terrorism cannot be fully answered without input from the intended recipients, the MMRS program communities themselves. The initial section of the following proposed survey, which could be administered at any point in the course of the contract or after the completion of the contract, solicits that input directly. It then goes on to query the respondent, whom the committee envisions as OEP's primary contact in the community, about the perceived abilities of the community in a number of functional areas that the committee believes are essential to preparedness. It concludes with several open-ended questions regarding the remaining barriers to preparedness for CBR terrorism and changes in the day-to-day and disaster-oriented operations of the public safety, public health, and health services agencies in the community.

SURVEY FOR MMRS PROGRAM CONTRACTORS

Part I

The Office of Emergency Preparedness provides guidance and assistance to its contractor cities through a variety of mechanisms. These are described on page 2 of this folder [page 2 is omitted from this IOM report, since the descriptions are included earlier in this chapter]. Please read the descriptions, and then, for each of the assistance mechanisms listed below, indicate by checking the appropriate boxes whether you were previously aware of it and, if sc, whether you found it helpful (a) in preparing the products ("deliverables") demanded by your contract and (b) in preparing your community to cope with chemical, biological, or radiological (CBR) terrorism.

		I was previously aware of this source of assistance, and **for meeting the terms of my contract**, I found it:				I was previously aware of this source of assistance, and **for preparing my community to cope with CBR terrorism**, I found it:			
ASSISTANCE	I was **NOT** aware of this assistance until now	Very useful	Useful	Not useful	Made the job more difficult	Very useful	Useful	Not useful	Made the job more difficult
"Planning considerations" for a bioterrorism plan	[ ]	[ ]	[ ]	[ ]	[ ]	[ ]	[ ]	[ ]	[ ]
Consultation with a regional project officer	[ ]	[ ]	[ ]	[ ]	[ ]	[ ]	[ ]	[ ]	[ ]
Consultation with OEP Headquarters	[ ]	[ ]	[ ]	[ ]	[ ]	[ ]	[ ]	[ ]	[ ]

continued

ASSISTANCE	I was **NOT** aware of this assistance until now	I was previously aware of this source of assistance, and **for meeting the terms of my contract**, I found it:				I was previously aware of this source of assistance, and **for preparing my community to cope with CBR terrorism**, I found it:			
		Very useful	Useful	Not useful	Made the job more difficult	Very useful	Useful	Not useful	Made the job more difficult
Yearly meeting of representatives from all MMRS program cities	[ ]	[ ]	[ ]	[ ]	[ ]	[ ]	[ ]	[ ]	[ ]
MMRS "track" at annual National Disaster Medical System (NDMS) meeting	[ ]	[ ]	[ ]	[ ]	[ ]	[ ]	[ ]	[ ]	[ ]
List of contacts for all MMRS program cities	[ ]	[ ]	[ ]	[ ]	[ ]	[ ]	[ ]	[ ]	[ ]
Public website	[ ]	[ ]	[ ]	[ ]	[ ]	[ ]	[ ]	[ ]	[ ]
Sample or model monthly report	[ ]	[ ]	[ ]	[ ]	[ ]	[ ]	[ ]	[ ]	[ ]
Completed plans from other cities	[ ]	[ ]	[ ]	[ ]	[ ]	[ ]	[ ]	[ ]	[ ]
OEP-funded research on common problem areas	[ ]	[ ]	[ ]	[ ]	[ ]	[ ]	[ ]	[ ]	[ ]

Checklist for self-evaluation of contract compliance	[ ]	[ ]	[ ]	[ ]	[ ]	[ ]	[ ]	[ ]	[ ]
Other OEP assistance (please describe below)	[ ]	[ ]	[ ]	[ ]	[ ]	[ ]	[ ]	[ ]	[ ]

Part II

Please help us assess the effectiveness of the MMRS program by rating your community's current ability to cope with the consequences of a CBR terrorism event (alone or in concert with neighboring communities and state and federal agencies), using a five-point scale to estimate capabilities in each of the listed areas and a three-point scale to estimate the contribution of the MMRS program:

	CAPABILITY					MMRS PROGRAM CONTRIBUTION		
FUNCTIONAL AREA	Very low	Low	Moderate	High	Very high	None	Small	Large
Command and control								
Notification and alert procedures								
Public affairs								
Provision of accurate and timely information to responders and caregivers								
Management and augmentation of transportation assets								
Management and augmentation of medical personnel								
Management and augmentation of medical supplies and equipment								
Legal issues and credentialing, patient tracking and record keeping								
Epidemiological services and support								

Laboratory support

Protection of treatment facilities and personnel

Mental health services

Activation of mutual-aid support from federal, state, and local emergency response agencies

FOR CHEMICAL AND OVERT RADIOLOGICAL INCIDENTS:

Detection and identification of the weapon material or agent

Extraction of victims

Administration of the appropriate antidote

Decontamination of victims at the site

Emergency medical care for victims before their transportation to a definitive medical care facility

Emergency medical transportation of the patients to area hospitals

Management of patients arriving at hospitals without prior field treatment, screening, or decontamination

continued

Part II (continued)

FUNCTIONAL AREA	CAPABILITY					MMRS PROGRAM CONTRIBUTION		
	Very low	Low	Moderate	High	Very high	None	Small	Large
Definitive medical care at hospitals or designated off-site treatment facilities								
Appropriate pharmaceuticals to care for up to 1,000 victims								
Equipment and supplies required to care for up to 1,000 victims								
Transportation of patients to distant treatment facilities via NDMS								
Mass-fatality management								
Environmental surety (decontamination of property and material for reentry or reuse)								
FOR BIOLOGICAL INCIDENTS:								
Early recognition of disease outbreaks								

Timely diagnosis and identification of agents on the threat list

Mass immunization or prophylaxis

Definitive medical care at hospitals or designated off-site treatment facilities (up to 100 victims)

Definitive medical care at hospitals or designated off-site treatment facilities (100 to 10,000 victims)

Definitive medical care at hospitals or designated off-site treatment facilities (more than 10,000 victims)

Transportation of patients to distant treatment facilities via NDMS

Mass fatality management (up to 100 victims)

Mass fatality management (100 to 10,000 victims)

Mass fatality management (more than 10,000 victims)

Environmental surety (decontamination of property and material for reentry or reuse)

continued

Part III

Please describe any changes in day-to-day operations of the public safety, public health, or health services agencies in your community that are attributable, in whole or in part, to your participation in the MMRS program.

Has your community suffered a disaster of any sort, natural or technological, since you began participating in the MMRS program? If so, please describe the disaster and the role, if any, that your MMRS or the planning and coordination required to develop an MMRS might have had on your community's ability to cope with that disaster.

Please list or describe any barriers, financial, political, cultural, or other, that hinder full preparedness in your community.

8

Feedback to Office of Emergency Preparedness on Program Success

Regardless of how the Metropolitan Medical Response System (MMRS) program is managed by the U.S. Department of Health and Human Services' Office of Emergency Preparedness (OEP), the ultimate test of the program's worth lies in how well it has helped local communities prepare for the consequences of a massive terrorist attack with chemical, biological, or radiological (CBR) weapons. The survey described in the previous chapter begins to answer this question by soliciting the opinions of the communities themselves. This chapter complements that approach by presenting the recommendations of the Committee on Evaluation of the Metropolitan Medical Response System Program for an independent and systematic assessment of the response capabilities of the large metropolitan areas that have or will participate in the MMRS program. The title to the chapter was chosen to emphasize an important assumption or guiding principle of the committee: that program assessment is primarily for the purpose of identifying and correcting shortfalls in OEP's MMRS program. Several other interrelated principles also underlie the chapter and the committee's recommendations:

- Evaluation should be part of a continuous learning and continuous quality improvement program, not a one-time snapshot. This implies a continuing relationship between the communities and their evaluators that includes financial as well as technical and educational support.
- "Preparedness" is a meaningless abstract concept, since threats vary among communities and change over time, perhaps even in response

to a community's level of preparedness; readiness should be seen as a process rather than a state.

- Preparedness requires not only numerous specific capabilities, typically the responsibilities of independent offices, agencies, and institutions, but also seamless coordination of those capabilities into a coherent response. The former may be envisioned as the teeth of a comb, the latter as the base or backbone of the comb.
- Information and the ability to acquire, process, and appropriately distribute it to essential sites and personnel are central to the effective management of critical incidents including terrorism in its many forms.
- Evaluation is an exercise designed to guide the distribution of local, state, and federal resources. Evaluations should be valued and understood as an opportunity for local communities to determine the areas in need of improvement and support rather than as a test of communities' self-reliance.
- Evaluation by OEP should be a multilevel process that includes (1) periodic review of documents and records, (2) observation of community-initiated exercises and drills, and (3) on-site assessment. The committee views the on-site assessment as comprising both interviews of individuals about specific capabilities and a scenario-driven group interaction focused on cooperation and coordination.
- A relatively small subset of the nearly 500 preparedness indicators identified in the Phase I report (Institute of Medicine, 2001) can be used to identify critical areas in need of improvement for a given community.

As noted earlier in the report, in the absence of any proper control cities or pre-MMRS data, it will be impossible to unequivocally assign credit to OEP for high states of preparedness. Most of the larger cities have received training and equipment from the U.S. Department of Defense or the U.S. Department of Justice, some have received grants and training from the Centers for Disease Control and Prevention (CDC), and all have spent time and money from state and local budgets. The MMRS program's emphasis on multiagency, multijurisdictional planning undoubtedly played a major role in increasing preparedness in many cities, but no large city could become well prepared solely as a result of the relatively meager funding provided by the OEP contracts.

The remainder of this chapter describes a three-element evaluation procedure built upon these principles. The three elements are review of written documents and data, a site visit by a team of peer reviewers, and observations at exercises and drills. The three procedures are complementary means of analyzing the community's response capabilities, and the next two sections focus on first identifying a subset of essential capabilities and then specifying preparedness criteria for each. The chapter concludes by proposing some specific procedures for gathering data at exercises and drills and at site visits.

ESSENTIAL RESPONSE CAPABILITIES

As noted above, the committee's Phase I report (Institute of Medicine, 2001) identified nearly 500 potential indicators of preparedness (see Appendix E). Chapter 6 provides information on how and why the committee arrived at these indicators, suggests that no evaluation would be likely to use all of the defined indicators, and proposes a means of beginning the selection problem, namely, to look first for output measures and to rely on process and input measures only when corresponding outputs are unavailable. This approach greatly reduces the number of potential items to be included in an evaluation effort, but the evaluator is still left with a large number of items. The committee has made further reductions by analyzing the critical actions required for effective responses to large-scale CBR terrorism incidents, that is, the essential response capabilities.

The specific characteristics and importance of these essential response capabilities vary with the type of agent and the other details of the incident, as do the relative importance of the various capabilities, but the many elements on the list of MMRS program contract deliverables and the corresponding preparedness indicators can be integrated into a list of 23 essential functions. They are listed below in the order in which they would generally become necessary:

1. Relationship development (Communication, coordination, and control are especially critical in responding to events like those of the autumn of 2001)

–city agencies, state and other local governments

–federal agencies and local federal facilities

–private institutions, especially health care institutions

–voluntary community organizations (e.g., Red Cross, churches, ham radio operators)

2. Communication system development

–telephonic, computer, and radio hardware; points of contact; procedures

–alternatives to commercial services, which are likely to be overwhelmed during a terrorist event.

–mutual aid pacts with nearby communities address compatible communication equipment

3. Hazard assessment

–high-risk sites identified and contingency plans developed (although OEP asks for plans for coping with 1000 victims of a chemical attack and 3 levels of biological attack, each community should use this assessment to make estimates of likely casualty volumes specific to the area and situation).

4. Training

–awareness, equipment, treatment, exercises

–fire and police departments, emergency medical technicians, emergency services and public health personnel, hospitals, individual medical care providers

5. Equipment and supplies

–purchase and maintenance (general purpose as well as specialized for CBR agents)

–reception and distribution of "push package" from CDC

6. Mass immunization and prophylaxis

7. Addressing the information needs of the public and the news media (Experience from September 11 and the anthrax incidents emphasizes the importance of early and frequent communication with the public through a single authoritative spokesperson on health matters.)

8. First responder protection

9. Rescue and stabilization of victims

10. Diagnosis and agent identification

–hardware and software to monitor health trends in close to real time

11. Decontamination of victims (at site of exposure or at a hospital or treatment site)

12. Transportation of victims

–from incident site to hospital or casualty collection point

–from hospital to hospital (including use of National Disaster Medical System [NDMS])

–patient tracking system

13. Distribution of supplies, equipment, and pharmaceuticals
–from local cache
–from National Pharmaceutical Stockpile

14. Shelter and feeding of evacuated and displaced persons
–provisions for emergency shelter for persons fleeing sites of perceived danger

15. Definitive medical care
–trained personnel, beds, supplies and equipment
–locations, in event that existing hospitals' capacities are inadequate
–mass immunization or distribution of drugs or vaccines

16. Mental health services for responders, victims, caregivers, and their families

17. Volunteer utilization and control

18. Crowd and traffic control
–at and near facilities rendering emergency medical care
–at hospitals or facilities dispensing medication
–along evacuation routes

19. Evacuation and quarantine decisions and operations

20. Fatality management
–large numbers of contaminated or infectious corpses

21. Environmental cleanup, physical restoration of facilities, and certification of safety

22. Follow-up study of responder, caregiver, and victim health

23. Process for continuous evaluation of needs and resources, during and after exercises and actual CBR, mass-casualty, and hazardous material (hazmat) events and disease outbreaks

With these 23 essential functions or capabilities as a guide, selection of a set of preparedness indicators for evaluation is considerably easier. The committee believes that the set of indicators described in the following section can serve as a suitable proxy for preparedness. Evaluating even this limited set of indicators nevertheless demands evaluators or auditors with diverse backgrounds and expertise in a variety of areas as well as several auditing techniques. The approach taken by the committee calls for a combination of evaluation of documents submitted to OEP by the community to be evaluated, on-site questioning by a site-visit team, and direct observation of drills and exercises.

PREPAREDNESS INDICATORS FOR EVALUATION OF WRITTEN SUBMISSIONS, ON-SITE INSPECTION, AND OBSERVED EXERCISES

Table 8-1 shows a list of preparedness indicators selected from the tables of Appendix E that cover the 23 essential MMRS capabilities outlined in the previous section. In accordance with the philosophy expressed at the beginning of this chapter, the committee sought to keep the number of indicators requiring on-site interviews or observations to a manageable number by selecting a number of indicators that involved documents or other written records that could be mailed or otherwise sent to the evaluators. For many essential capabilities, such written records were the optimal or only feasible indicators; in other cases, selection of a written evaluation rather than an on-site evaluation was a compromise between the optimal measure and the realities of time and expense for both the assessor and the assessed. As suggested in Chapter 6, the committee considers output indicators more likely to be valid than process and input indicators, and Table 8-1 therefore heavily favors output indicators for on-site evaluations. Should any of the listed output indicators be unavailable, the committee expects the evaluator to use the corresponding process or input indicators to guide a judgment about preparedness.

PREPAREDNESS CRITERIA

No generally agreed-upon model for local preparedness exists, nor are good data or even a solid consensus available about what constitutes acceptable objective evidence of capability for most of the preparedness indicators listed above. The committee is also sensitive to the great diversity of circumstances facing the nation's cities and the variety of ways in which they are organized to respond to emergencies. The committee therefore chose not to try to specify rigid standards for each of the countless possible combinations of incident types and response approaches. Instead, the proposed assessment program puts considerable faith in the judgment of what is now a relatively small but rapidly growing cadre of individuals who have been in the forefront of responding to and planning for responses to incidents related to the use of CBR agents. Nevertheless, to ensure the comparabilities of the assessments made by different evaluators and to provide communities with some indication of what those experts will be looking for, the committee has assembled below, for each of the essential capabilities listed in Table 8-1, criteria that should serve as the core of evaluators' judgments about preparedness. Armed with these criteria, it should be possible for an evaluator or a team of evaluators to determine whether a community is well prepared, prepared, or poorly prepared in each of the 23 essential capabilities. The committee feels strongly that the real value in the proposed evaluation system lies in identifying capabilities in need of improvement, and has therefore resisted the temptation to specify a passing grade. The fact is that, as noted on page 113, preparedness as an abstract concept is meaningless. That is, even a perfect score on each of the 23 capabilities will not guarantee an optimal response to all imaginable CBR events; less than a perfect score makes it easy to imagine an event that will be handled poorly.

1. Relationship Development (Partnering)

Preparedness Indicator

Documentation of effective coordination in an exercise or an actual incident with or without CBR agents.

- The lead agency provides written documentation of an MMRS-wide response system that includes management, operations, logistics, planning and intelligence, and finance and administration activities.
- The lead agency provides a list of community-level response plans used regularly for non-terrorist-related emergencies or disasters, for example:
    - Emergency Operations Plan
    - Multiple Casualty Incident Plan
    - Hazmat Response Plan
    - Emergency Medical Service (EMS) Management Plan
- The lead agency provides an after-action report from a full-scale exercise, which should be conducted at least once every 3 years.
- The lead agency documents actual events, including evaluation of potential for terrorism by the incident commander.

Preparedness Indicator

Evidence from exercises or actual events demonstrating workable interface among local plans.

TABLE 8-1 Preparedness Indicators and Mode of Evaluation of MMRS Plan Elements Relevant to Each of 23 Essential Capabilities

Essential Capability	MMRS Plan Element
1. Relationship development (partnering)	**2.02** Description of how responses to a CBR terrorism incident by public safety, public health, and health services sectors will be coordinated
	3.04 Coordination with other political, mutual-aid, or other MMRS program jurisdictions
2 Communication system development	**3.07** Detailed notification and alert procedures via redundant systems
	3.09 Provisions for accurate and timely dissemination of information among MMRS members
	8.01 Procedures for notification of hospitals, clinics, health maintenance organizations (HMOs), etc., that an incident has occurred
	8.New 1 Procedures for recall of staff
3. Hazard assessment	**2.New 1** Description of the planning environment (i.e., identification of local hazards, baseline strengths, vulnerabilities)
4. Training	**3.20** A schedule for exercises
	9.01 Training requirements for all personnel responding to the scene of an incident or providing care to victims of a CBR agent-related incident

Preparedness Indicator	Written	Site Visit	Drill
Documentation of effective coordination in an exercise or an actual incident with or without CBR agents	X		X
Evidence from exercises or actual events demonstrating workable interface among local plans	X	X	X
• Documented success by regular testing or during actual use in an emergency	X		X
• System is not dependent on commercial services alone.	X	X	
• Mutual aid agreements with surrounding communities insure interoperability of key communication systems	X		
Demonstration of effective use of all systems in periods of peak demand through unannounced tests or use in an actual emergency	X		X
• Percentage of facilities contacted in 1 hour during weekly notification checks	X		
• Time from initial contact to initiation of hospital disaster plan or incident command system	X		X
• Calls to random sample of list demonstrate that list is up to date		X	
• Percentage of staff returning calls in 2 hours	X		X
A communitywide assessment identifies strengths, barriers and challenges, and a priority list for planning efforts	X		
Collection of after-action reports	X		
• Demonstration of knowledge of subject matter to peer reviewer by selected sample of trained personnel from any level of any participating organizations or through functional drills, communitywide exercises, or responses to actual CBR agent, hazmat, or infectious disease outbreak events		X	X
• Certification or other nationally recognized affirmation of CBR agent-specific knowledge and skills, if such means for certification become available in the future	X		

TABLE 8-1 Continued

Essential Capability	MMRS Plan Element
5. Equipment and supplies	**10.02** Quantities of pharmaceuticals sufficient to care for 1,000 victims of a chemical agent and for entire affected population for 24 hours after a biological incident
	10.04 Detailed procedures for equipment maintenance and pharmaceutical storage
6 Mass immunization or prophylaxis	**7.05** New plans or augmentation of existing plans for management and implementation of a mass immunization or prophylaxis plan
7. Attention to the information needs of the public and the news media	**3.08** Detailed management procedures for public affairs
8. First responder protection	**5.11** Procedures for procurement and provision of appropriate equipment and supplies
	8.05 Availability of adequate personal protective equipment for hospital and clinic providers

Preparedness Indicator	Written	Site Visit	Drill
Availability of all required antidotes, antibiotics, and immune sera, in appropriate quantities, for inspection by site-visit team or peer reviewer		X	
• Evidence that the mechanism of delivery and storage is secure in natural disasters, mock drills, earthquakes, or hazmat events		X	
• Consistency of inventory with records of pharmacy and therapeutics committee meetings	X		
• Knowledge of procedures for return of unused supplies and decontamination of equipment by logistics personnel		X	
• Evidence that a sample of equipment selected by peer reviewer is in working order		X	
• Performance of required maintenance and/or prompt retrieval of maintenance manual by logistics personnel when queried by peer reviewer		X	
• After-action report detailing successful response to a CBR incident (real or a hoax), a natural outbreak of disease (e.g., a meningitis or influenza vaccination campaign or an outbreak of rabies or giardiasis), or a large-scale exercise	X		
• Identification in the plan of distribution sites and required personnel	X		
• Percentage of responder and caregiving personnel immunized if the plan calls for prophylactic immunizations	X		
• A knowledgeable and credible spokesperson has been designated to provide health information to the public in the event of a terrorist attack with a CBR agent.	X		
• Collection of finished communiqués	X		
• Documented use of media packages in CBR agent-related hoaxes or incidents or other hazmat-related or epidemic events	X		
Demonstration that the appropriate types and quantities of equipment and supplies have been purchased and are readily accessible		X	X
Demonstration of competency with equipment (e.g., by a respirator fit test) for expert peer reviewer		X	X

TABLE 8-1 Continued

Essential Capability	MMRS Plan Element
9. Rescue and stabilization of victims	**5.03** Detailed procedures for extraction of victims from event site
	5.04 Detailed procedures for administration of appropriate antidote
	5.06 Procedures for victim triage and initial care before transport to definitive medical care facility
	8.03 Provisions for the capability of local health care facilities to provide triage and initiate definitive care
10. Diagnosis and agent identification	**5.02** Detailed procedures for detection and identification of agents
	7.03 Identification of early-warning indicators that will be used to alert local officials of a bioterrorism event
	8.07 Ability of medical staff to recognize and treat casualties caused by CBR agents
11. Decontamination of victims	**5.05** Detailed procedures for decontamination of victims
	5.09 Procedures for management of patients arriving at hospitals without prior field screening or decontamination

Preparedness Indicator	Written	Site Visit	Drill
Hands-on demonstration (for peer reviewer or in a large-scale drill or actual hazmat incident) of safe and efficient extraction of a victim from a contaminated area		X	X
Hands-on demonstration (for peer reviewer or in a large-scale drill or actual hazmat incident) of administration of proper antidote		X	X
Hands-on demonstration (for peer reviewer or in a large-scale drill or actual hazmat incident) of victim triage and initial care		X	X
• Numbers, types, and durations of diversions in previous 3 months	X		
• Numbers and types of patients transferred out of the hospital to other facilities in previous 3 months	X		
Hands-on demonstration (for peer reviewer or in a large-scale drill or actual hazmat incident) of agent detection and identification		X	X
• Demonstration of appropriate use of early-warning indicators in peer-review interview, exercise, or actual event		X	X
• Percentage of laboratory personnel certified by relevant professional organization	X		
• Demonstration to peer reviewer of knowledge and availability of supplies to carry out specified assays or successful detection of a test sample containing a close relative of the designated agents		X	X
• Laboratory quality assurance test results	X		
• Demonstration of knowledge in responses to peer reviewer questions, exercise, or actual event		X	X
• Hands-on demonstration (for peer reviewer or in a large-scale drill or actual hazmat incident) of decontamination of victims		X	X
• List of all required equipment on hand or readily accessible	X		
• Actual decontamination of individual patients	X		
• Successful decontamination of multiple patients in an exercise or actual hazmat event	X		X

TABLE 8-1 Continued

Essential Capability	MMRS Plan Element
	8.02 Procedures for protection of hospitals, clinics, and HMOs from contamination from environmental or patient sources (lockdown procedures)
12. Transportation of victims	**3.11** Provisions for control of transportation assets, medical and nonmedical
	5.07 Provisions for emergency medical transportation of victims
	4.01 Detailed procedures for preparation of patients for movement to other areas of the region or nation
13. Distribution of supplies, equipment, and pharmaceuticals	**10.New 1** Procedures for distributing pharmaceuticals and equipment to local personnel and facilities
	10.New 2 Procedures for requesting, receiving, and distributing pharmaceuticals from the National Pharmaceutical Stockpile (NPS)
	8.New 2 Procedures for delivery of nonmedical supplies

Preparedness Indicator	Written	Site Visit	Drill
• Numbers of secondary infections of staff or other patients in prior 6 months	X		
• Current conversion rate for positive tuberculosis (purified protein derivative) skin tests among staff	X		
• Numbers of negative-pressure isolation rooms available, overall and in emergency departments (EDs)	X		
• Numbers of tuberculosis, rubella, or varicella patients admitted to nonisolation rooms in prior 6 months	X		
• Numbers of staff furloughed due to exposure to patients with varicella, rubella, or other infectious diseases in prior 6 months	X		
• For the most recent tuberculosis patient, the time from examination to the time of isolation	X		
Availability of anticipated assets on short notice for random check, planned exercise, or actual emergency	X		X
Availability and response times in exercises or actual mass-casualty events	X		X
• Awareness of plan and procedures and when and how to initiate them by emergency medical services and hospital officials		X	
• Evidence of NDMS support for MMRS program plan and procedures for activation	X		X
Evidence from drill, actual event, or questioning by expert peer reviewer that local distribution of MMRS program pharmaceuticals and equipment will be rapid enough to maintain local supplies for at least the initial 24 hours of an event	X	X	X
Evidence from drill, actual event, or questioning by expert peer reviewer that local distribution of NPS supplies (push packages and vender-managed inventory) will be rapid enough to maintain local supplies after initial 24 hours of an event	X	X	X
• No disruption of services due to shortages during a drill or mass-casualty event	X		X
• Response times for deliveries	X		
• Demonstration that an alternative supplier has necessary quantities or can deliver them in 24 hours	X	X	

TABLE 8-1 Continued

Essential Capability	MMRS Plan Element
14. Shelter and feeding of evacuated and displaced persons	Not addressed in contracts
15. Definitive medical care	**3.12** Detailed procedures for the management and augmentation of medical personnel
	8.01 Procedures for notification of hospitals, clinics, HMOs, etc., that an incident has occurred
	8.06 Local availability of adequate pharmaceuticals and equipment (ventilators) or plans to obtain them in a timely manner
	8.07 Ability of medical staff to recognize and treat casualties caused by CBR agents

Preparedness Indicator	Written	Site Visit	Drill
• Demonstration that a lead agency responsible for evacuee shelter and feeding has been identified and has been demonstrated to have effective working relationships with leadership for fire and police departments, public health agencies, emergency management agencies, and other voluntary agencies that provide evacuee shelter and feeding (e.g., demonstration that the local chapter of the American Red Cross has a working relationship with the Salvation Army)	X		X
• Demonstration that the lead agency's disaster plan reflects special standard operating procedures for sheltering evacuees of CBR agent-related incidents	X		
Demonstration of effective use of all communication systems, at multiple sites and for several types of medical personnel, in periods of peak demand, through unannounced tests or use in an actual emergency (snowstorm, hurricane, etc.)	X		
• Documented resolution of any issues related to cross-jurisdictional licensure and liability coverage	X		X
• Percentage of facilities contacted in 1 hour during weekly notification checks	X		
• Time from initial contact to initiation of hospital disaster plan or incident command system	X	X	X
• Availability of all essential antidotes, antibiotics, and immune sera, in appropriate quantities, for inspection by site-visit team or peer reviewer		X	
• Evidence of effective collaboration in coping with recent national shortages of influenza and tetanus vaccines and gamma globulin and shortages of antibiotics during emergencies	X		
• Response time to retrieve requested items in drills or in actual cases	X		X
• Laboratory quality assurance test results	X		
• Demonstration of knowledge in responses to peer-reviewer questions, exercise, or actual event		X	X
• Certification or other nationally recognized affirmation of CBR agent-specific knowledge and skills, if such means for certification become available in the future	X		
• Time from examination of tuberculosis patients to isolation	X		
• Number and type of negative-pressure isolation rooms available in EDs and in total	X	X	

TABLE 8-1 Continued

Essential Capability	MMRS Plan Element
16 Mental health services for responders, victims, caregivers, and their families	**3.22** Designation of mental health care for emergency workers, victims and their families, and others in community needing special assistance
17. Volunteer utilization and control	Not addressed in contracts
1.8 Crowd and traffic control	**3.18** Provisions for crowd control
	3.19 Provisions for protection of treatment facilities and personnel
19 Evacuation and quarantine decisions, operations	Not addressed in contracts

Preparedness Indicator	Written	Site Visit	Drill
After-action reports from other kinds of disasters or exercises that document coordination, availability, use, and effectiveness of mental health professionals	X		
• Demonstration that the lead voluntary agency maintains inventory of trained volunteers for mental and physical health, family services, and other purposes	X		
• Demonstration that the lead voluntary agency responds to disaster events within 2 hours of notification; this response includes shelter, feeding, disaster-related health services, disaster-related mental health services, damage assessment, and family services, as appropriate.	X		
• Demonstration that "spontaneous" volunteers are effectively screened, oriented and trained, given identification, and deployed	X		
• Demonstration that the language and the demography and culture of the communities that the volunteers serve are kept in mind when the volunteers are selected and trained		X	
• Demonstration that an established plan provides for crowd control at special events or during civil disturbances	X		
• Demonstration that officers receive regular training for these responsibilities	X		
• Demonstration that adequate protective equipment is available for police officers	X		
After-action reports that document crowd and traffic control at events with large attendances such as sporting events, concerts, and political conventions and/or in prior natural or technological disasters	X		
• Written plan that includes procedures for deciding upon and conducting public safety measures such as shelter in place, orderly evacuation, quarantine of individuals and geographical areas, and isolation of patients or groups of patients.	X		
• Demonstration that the identified leadership can verbalize the contents of the procedure to evacuate a contaminated facility		X	
• Demonstration that the identified leadership can verbalize the contents of the procedure to initiate isolation or quarantine		X	

TABLE 8-1 Continued

Essential Capability	MMRS Plan Element
20. Fatality management	**7.10** Procedures for augmentation of morgue facilities and staff
	7.11 Procedures for decontamination or isolation of human remains
21. Environmental cleanup, physical restoration of facilities, and certification of safety	**7.12** Procedures for identification of environmental risk and determination of the need for decontamination or vector intervention
	7.13 A process for safe reentry into the affected area in consultation with local, state, and federal environmental agencies
22. Follow-up study of responder, caregiver, and victim health	Not addressed in contract
23. Process for continuous evaluation of needs and resources	**3.21** Assignment of responsibility for after-action reports and addressing report findings

Preparedness Indicator	Written	Site Visit	Drill
• Contingency contracts or other arrangements for storage capacity with local hospital morgues, mortuaries, warehouses, other facilities with cold-storage capabilities, and sources of refrigerated trucks	X		
• Evidence of NDMS support and procedures for activation (joint training, tabletop demonstration of interface with Disaster Mortuary Operational Response Teams)	X		
• Hands-on demonstration of decontamination in an exercise or actual incident			X
• Evidence that standard operating procedures are available at morgue facilities in sufficient quantity to distribute to any expedient sites and that required personnel is available		X	
Demonstration of an effective process to expert peer reviewer; in response to questioning or by performance in an exercise, actual hazmat event, or disease outbreak		X	X
Same as above for MMRS Plan Element 7.12			
Demonstration that the response plan includes practical process for scientific investigation of human health effects in responders, caregivers, and victims, and evidence that baseline data on employees are available	X		
• Possession by all participating agencies and institutions of a collection of after-action reports		X	
• During-action reports from extended exercises or prolonged responses to actual CBR agent or hazmat events	X		
• Evidence for changes in structure or functioning in response to deficiencies identified in after-action or during-action reports	X		

- A legally constituted mutual-aid plan includes members of all professions participating in the MMRS.
- The lead agency documents mutual aid during actual events that involve the community's personnel (non-terrorist-related or routine events).
- The lead agency provides a plan for receiving outside assistance from the coroner or medical examiner, hospitals, and the public health department (this may include a state-level mutual-aid plan, preidentified federal resource, or professional organization-based plans).

2. Communication System Development

Preparedness Indicator

Documented success of notification and alert procedures by regular testing or during actual use in an emergency.

- A notification plan provides an immediate alert to all agencies, hospitals, and other entities with an essential or important role in MMRS response.
- An activity log shows that testing is being conducted at least weekly and at random times, including nights and weekends.
- An activity log shows an 80 percent response rate during testing (at least weekly) or during an actual emergency.

Preparedness Indicator

Demonstration of accurate and timely dissemination of information among MMRS members by all communications systems in periods of peak demand through unannounced tests or use in an actual emergency.

- The lead agency demonstrates the availability of a system that disseminates timely (within minutes) information to MMRS members.
- An activity log demonstrates regular use of the notification system for information dissemination for weather and other recurring events (for example, diversion of patients to other hospitals or hospital closures).
- An activity log shows an 80 percent response rate, confirming receipt of information by recipients.
- The lead agency provides evidence that two-way communications are in place, for example, that hospitals are reporting ED closures, with the compiled data being distributed back to hospitals in near real time.

Preparedness Indicator

System is not dependent on commercial services alone.

Preparedness Indicator

Mutual aid agreements with surrounding communities insure interoperability of key communication systems (compatible hardware, common radio frequencies, cross-training)

Preparedness Indicator

Time from initial contact to initiation of hospital disaster plan or incident command system.

- One or more hospitals demonstrate that operational incident management is in place within 20 minutes of notification.
- One or more hospitals demonstrate that hospital emergency operations are being implemented at the operational level (operational personnel are implementing their assignments) within 5 minutes of notification.

3. Hazard Assessment

Preparedness Indicator

A communitywide assessment identifies strengths, barriers and challenges, and a priority list for planning efforts.

- Sources of information are reported and appropriate (i.e., what is basis of preparation?).
- All relevant institutions (health officers, laboratory personnel, hazmat personnel, etc.) have participated in the assessment.
- Criteria for prioritization are explicit (e.g., is a high likelihood of occurrence or an event with a large impact weighted more heavily?).
- A variety of potential CBR scenarios have been considered.
- The rationale for the assets needed to respond to different hazards is explicit and reasonable.
- Estimates of potential numbers of casualties have been related to types and circumstances of hazard exposure.

4. Training

Preparedness Indicator

A collection of after-action reports documents a program of drills and exercises.

- Tabletop exercises should be performed with senior police and fire personnel at least every 3 years.
- A full-scale MMRS-wide exercise should be conducted at least every 3 years.

Preparedness Indicator

Demonstration of knowledge of subject matter by MMRS personnel from several levels and several organizations (also, see the discussion of preparedness indicators under the elements Diagnosis and Agent Identification and Definitive Medical Care below).

- Eighty percent of selected MMRS personnel correctly answer at least 80 percent of questions on a multiple-choice test of recognition indicators and response precautions for a terrorist event.
- Terrorism awareness training is provided in police and fire academy training.
- Hazmat training for retention of certification is provided for all hazmat team members.
- Refresher training in CBR agent recognition and response is given to all police, fire, EMS, and Office of Emergency Services personnel at least every 3 years.
- Command training (at the fire chief or police captain academy) includes a terrorism element (this can also be done through a tabletop exercise).

5. Equipment and Supplies

Preparedness Indicator

Availability of all required antidotes, antibiotics, and immune sera, in appropriate quantities, for inspection by site-visit team or peer reviewer.

- An inventory lists all pharmaceuticals required by MMRS medical protocols.

- Calculations or mathematical models for estimating the needs of the region's population are available.
- The property officer can demonstrate updating of the system by analysis of the entire stock.
- The property officer can demonstrate the mechanism used to analyze the stock at other supply sites.
- Written protocols cover the movement of materials from site to site.
- Links to central resources (from the state or CDC) for supplies such as immune sera (e.g., botulinum antitoxin) and variola virus vaccine or immunoglobulin can be demonstrated.

Preparedness Indicator

Evidence that the mechanism of delivery and storage is secure in natural disasters, mock drills, earthquakes, or hazmat events.

- Supplies are available at more than a single storage site.
- Records of controlled drugs are complete and up to date.
- Storage site personnel are familiar with procedures for the release of supplies and equipment and the documentation of their release.

Preparedness Indicator

The inventory is consistent with the records of the pharmacy and therapeutics committee meetings.

Preparedness Indicator

Logistics personnel are familiar with procedures for the return of unused supplies and decontamination of equipment for restorage and reuse.

Preparedness Indicator

Demonstration that a sample of equipment selected by the peer reviewer is in working order.

Preparedness Indicator

Performance of required maintenance or prompt retrieval of maintenance manual by logistics personnel when queried by the peer reviewer.

- A biomedical engineer has checked equipment upon its receipt.
- User operation and maintenance training has been conducted if the equipment is not similar to or compatible with that used in the local hospitals and by EMSs.
- The maintenance log is available and up to date.

6. Mass Immunization and Prophylaxis

Preparedness Indicator

An after-action report detailing a successful response to a natural outbreak of disease, an incident (real or a hoax) involving a CBR agent, or a large-scale exercise. The report includes the following:

- the method by which the index case was identified;
- the time frame between onset and identification of the agent involved;
- verification of reporting of the agent involved to the local public health system,
- a chronology of the investigation;
- the identification of the professionals and agencies involved;
- the roles and responsibilities of the professionals and agencies involved; and
- a summary of the activity, the actions taken, and recommendations for improvement.

Preparedness Indicator

A plan that identifies distribution sites and required personnel, that recognizes the importance of essential public safety personnel and health care providers, and that encompasses site security and record keeping.

- The community has a well-defined public immunization effort through the local health department, hospital, or community collaborative.
- The responsible entity can identify the percentage of all immunizations given in the community that are provided through the public program.
- The responsible entity has a record-keeping system that identifies community providers who administer vaccines received through the public health system to low-income patients.
- An electronic immunization registry that includes public and private vaccine providers is in place.

Preparedness Indicator

The percentage of responder and caregiving personnel who have been immunized if the plan calls for prophylactic immunizations.

- The lead agency can document that at least 80 percent of designated personnel have been immunized.

7. Attention to the Information Needs of the Public and the News Media

Preparedness Indicator

A knowledgeable and credible spokesperson has been designated to provide health information to the public in the event of a terrorist attack with a CBR agent.

Preparedness Indicator

A collection of finished communiqués.

- Basic press releases on chemical and biological threat agents are readily accessible in paper and electronic formats and in languages other than English if necessary to meet community needs.
- An Emergency Public Information plan applicable to all hazards is written.
- Trained public information officers with 24-hour call-back and contact information have been designated.
- All public information officers have basic awareness of issues related to terrorism.
- Library of resources related to CBR agents are available for public information offices, for example, *Jane's Manual,* the green book and the blue or red book of the U.S. Department of Defense or similar publications, articles from the *Journal of the American Medical Association,* websites, and other reference books.
- A media contact list is preloaded onto a broadcast fax machine or computer and includes contacts for television, radio, print media, and non-English-language publications.
- Emergency planners should anticipate the need to provide accurate information to victims' families through Web sites and patient locator systems that are created in advance and activated immediately following a catastrophic event.

Preparedness Indicator

Documented use of media packages in CBR agent-related hoaxes or incidents, other hazmat events, or disease outbreaks.

8. First Responder Protection

Preparedness Indicator

Appropriate types and quantities of personal protective equipment and supplies have been purchased and are readily accessible to both traditional first responders and hospital and clinic staff.

- The amounts and locations of the personal protective equipment that have been procured are consistent with the MMRS planning document's presumed incident size and methodology for determination of equipment needs.
- Inspection of at least two sites confirms the presence of the equipment specified in the inventory. Equipment should be readily accessible and clearly labeled at a site with appropriate temperature and humidity controls.
- Emergency and security staffs have immediate access to personal protective equipment.
    - The equipment is stored in an area without a lock.
    - If the equipment is stored in a locked area, staff can locate the key without assistance.
- On-duty personnel should be able to put on a breathing apparatus (e.g., masks or respirators) without coaching. Respiratory fit test (e.g., with banana oil or peppermint oil) should confirm that the breathing apparatus seals completely.
- On-duty personnel should be able to put on chemical protective apparel without coaching. When suited, personnel should be heavily sprayed with water to show that the suit excludes outside elements (i.e., to show that no water penetrates the body suit).

9. Rescue and Stabilization of Victims

Preparedness Indicator

Hands-on demonstration (for peer reviewer or in a large-scale drill or actual hazmat incident) of safe and efficient extraction of a victim from a contaminated area.

- Appropriate level of personal protective equipment is correctly worn and maintained by all personnel while they are in areas that may be contaminated with a CBR agent ("hot" and "warm" zones).
- Patients can be moved in a manner that is safe both for the patient

(e.g., spinal immobilization if the patient has received a trauma) and for the rescuer (e.g., the rescuer is able to correctly lift the patient with no compromise of his or her personal protective equipment).

Preparedness Indicator

Hands-on demonstration (for peer reviewer or in a large-scale drill or actual hazmat incident) of administration of proper antidote.

- Antidotes are packaged for operational deployment.
- Staff is able to deploy antidotes, distribute and administer antidotes in a timely fashion during a drill, or explain during a tabletop scenario how antidote distribution and administration would occur.

Preparedness Indicator

Hands-on demonstration (for peer reviewer or in a large-scale drill or actual hazmat incident) of victim triage and initial care.

- Triage rules and any variations in mass-casualty situations are well understood by both prehospital emergency medical and ED personnel.
- Data on numbers, types, and durations of ED diversions in previous 3 months demonstrate the consistent availability of emergency care for a wide variety of patients.

10. Diagnosis and Agent Identification

Preparedness Indicator

Hands-on demonstration (for peer reviewer or in a large-scale drill or actual hazmat incident) of chemical agent detection and identification.

Preparedness Indicator

Demonstration of appropriate use of early-warning indicators of epidemic disease in a peer-review interview, exercise, or actual event.

- Baseline data are available from a variety of sources.
- A designated individual or office monitors data on a daily basis.
- Decision rules and points of contact are available in the event of the discovery of unusual data points.
- The communication network allows the rapid dissemination of information among health officers, clinical laboratories, health care facilities, and practitioners.

Preparedness Indicator

Demonstration to peer reviewer by laboratory personnel of knowledge and availability of supplies to carry out specified assays or successful detection of a test sample containing a close relative of the designated agents.

- Laboratory quality assurance test results document capability to identify key CBR agents
- Laboratory personnel are certified by the relevant professional organization.

Preparedness Indicator

Simulated patients presenting to two or three area EDs with signs and symptoms of smallpox are diagnosed accurately and are effectively isolated, ED and hospital infection control practices are effected immediately, appropriate staff and community officials are notified, and appropriate supportive care is arranged as needed. (Hospitals must be warned that simulated patients of some sort may be a part of the site visit.)

11. Decontamination of Victims

Preparedness Indicator

Hands-on demonstration (for peer reviewer or in a large-scale drill or actual hazmat incident) of decontamination of victims at an incident site.

- Review the MMRS plan to identify required decontamination equipment and bases for choice of type and quantity.
    - The equipment chosen is adequate to support decontamination of up to 1,000 victims of a terrorist incident involving chemical agents.
- Inspection of at least one site confirms that the equipment is in inventory and is readily accessible.
    - The on-site inventory complies with the plan.
    - If the equipment is stored in a locked area, staff can locate the key without assistance.
- The necessary equipment can be set up and functioning within 30 minutes of arrival on site.
    - Procedures are in place for expedient decontamination and keeping ambulatory victims on site for 30 minutes.
    - Equipment setup is not dependent solely on members of the hazmat unit.
    - The training required for both setup and operation has been pro-

vided to enough personnel to ensure the capability of equipment operation at all times (24 hours a day, 7 days a week, every day of the year).

- Procedures and equipment will allow decontamination of at least 500 persons per hour.
  - An exercise processes mock ambulatory victims at a rate of at least 9 persons per minute.
- Procedures are applicable in all weather and all seasons.
  - The available cover, heating, and clean dry clothing are sufficient to protect ambulatory victims against hypothermia.

Preparedness Indicator

Actual decontamination of individual patients arriving at hospitals without prior field screening or decontamination or successful decontamination of multiple patients in an exercise or actual hazmat event.

- The decontamination system allows self-decontamination by ambulatory patients within minutes.
- The lead agency provides evidence that security personnel and triage nurses at hospital entry areas have been trained to recognize potentially contaminated patients and to prevent their entry into the facility.
- A drill provides evidence that multiple patients presenting simultaneously for decontamination can be adequately organized and managed (as determined by expert judgment).
- An appropriate CBR agent simulant is completely removed during a full decontamination exercise.

Preparedness Indicator

Effective procedures are in place to inhibit transmission of infectious disease within hospitals, clinics, and other treatment sites.

- No instance of secondary infections of staff or other patients in prior 6 months has been found.
- No conversions to positive tuberculosis skin tests have been detected among staff in the prior 6 months.
- Isolation rooms are available, in the ED and other departments.
- No tuberculosis, rubella, or varicella patients have been admitted to nonisolation rooms in the prior 6 months.
- No staff have been furloughed due to exposure to patients with varicella, rubella, or other infectious diseases in prior 6 months.
- For the most recent tuberculosis patient, the time from the examination to patient isolation has been less than 1 hour.

12. Transportation of Victims

Preparedness Indicator

List of available sources of vehicles and drivers for use in mass-casualty event, including those available through mutual-aid agreements, state agencies, and local federal facilities.

- The lead agency provides current contracts and other agreements with public and private entities for emergency transport (buses, vans, and trucks).
- The lead agency provides evidence of periodic communication with managers of anticipated transportation assets.
- Standard operating procedures reflect state laws and local policies.

Preparedness Indicator

Interviews with one EMS contracted emergency medical transport provider, one noncontracted medical transport provider, and one nonmedical transport agency to confirm knowledge of MMRS plan, including the circumstances in which personal protective equipment and decontamination of patient transport vehicles are required and the means of acquiring both.

Preparedness Indicator

Availability of anticipated transportation assets on short notice for random check, planned exercise, or actual mass-casualty emergency.

Preparedness Indicator

Awareness of plan and procedures for movement of patients to other areas of the region or nation by EMS and hospital officials and when and how to initiate them.

- Two hospital officials and an EMS official satisfy the site-visit interviewer if a previous exercise has not demonstrated knowledge of the MMRS plan and procedures.
- The lead agency provides evidence of NDMS support for the MMRS plan and procedure for activation.

13. Distribution of Supplies, Equipment, and Pharmaceuticals

Preparedness Indicator

Evidence from drill, actual event, or questioning by expert peer reviewer that local distribution of MMRS program pharmaceuticals and equipment will be rapid enough to maintain local supplies for at least the initial 24 hours of an event.

- EMS and hospital systems understand the predetermined protocol in the plan for the distribution of pharmaceuticals, supplies, and equipment, including:
  - the quantity and type of supplies and equipment available,
  - the locations of the primary and secondary storage sites,
  - the need for 24-hour accessibility to all storage sites,
  - the priorities for distribution,
  - the person who has the authority to order and distribute supplies and equipment,
- the means of transport of supplies and equipment to affected sites, and
- the means by which trained staff at the affected sites are to receive and use the equipment.

Preparedness Indicator

Evidence from drill, actual event, or questioning by expert peer reviewer that local distribution of National Pharmaceutical Stockpile (NPS) supplies will be rapid enough to maintain local supplies after the initial 24 hours of an event.

- EMS, hospital systems, and responsible local or state officials understand the predetermined plan for requesting, receiving, and distributing NPS supplies, whether they are from push packages or the vendor-maintained inventory, including:
  - the chain of command for requesting NPS supplies,
  - the quantity and type of pharmaceuticals available,
  - the plan for receiving NPS supplies and the availability of personnel to repackage NPS supplies for distribution to affected sites,
  - the transportation of NPS supplies to affected sites,
  - the distribution of NPS supplies to affected hospitals, and
  - the receipt and use of NPS supplies by appropriate personnel at the sites receiving the supplies.

Preparedness Indicator

No disruption of services due to shortages of nonmedical supplies during a drill or mass-casualty event.

- The hospital emergency command center has access to a list of primary suppliers and alternative suppliers for the following: fuel and utilities, laundry, foodstuffs, water, waste removal.
  - If the list is maintained outside the command center, command center staff demonstrate the availability of a nontelephone communication system for the exchange of information.
  - If the list is maintained outside the command center, command center staff demonstrate the ability to access those with information outside the usual work hours from 9 a.m. to 5 p.m., Monday through Friday.
- Hospitals can identify alternative hospital suppliers located within a 200-mile radius of the hospital. (Note that 200 miles is an arbitrary distance; an alternative distance could be selected, but the distance selected must allow delivery within 24 hours.)
- Hospital logistics personnel are familiar with the procedures of the local police or sheriff department for allowing suppliers to enter "sealed" areas.
  - The police or sheriff department has an up-to-date list of primary and alternative hospital suppliers.
- Hospitals have "standing emergency orders" with suppliers that the suppliers will automatically implement without contact from the hospitals.
  - Primary and alternative suppliers maintain at least a 48-hour inventory stock for normal demand.

14. Shelter and Feeding of Evacuated and Displaced Individuals

Preparedness Indicator

The lead agency responsible for evacuee shelter and feeding has been identified and has demonstrated effective working relationships with leadership of the fire and police departments, public health agencies, emergency management agencies, and other voluntary agencies that provide evacuee shelter and feeding (e.g., the local chapter of the American Red Cross has a working relationship with the Salvation Army).

- The agency demonstrates the capabilities to ensure the provision of food and shelter for its affected population and to ensure the feeding of emergency workers.

- The lead agency demonstrates the capability to feed and shelter 10 percent of its affected population (assuming an affected population of 25,000 to 50,000 people) and all emergency workers.
- The agency has an up-to-date list of buildings (e.g., schools) that have agreed to serve as shelters (as determined from an on-site review of documentation).
- The agency can demonstrate how quickly during exercises shelters can be set up and other essential participants notified (as determined by questioning by the interviewer on site).

Preparedness Indicator

The lead agency's disaster plan reflects special operating procedures for sheltering evacuees in scenarios involving CBR agents.

- The plan describes where and how evacuees will be decontaminated if necessary before they enter shelters and who will do the decontamination.
- The plan describes alternatives to sheltering evacuees if necessary because of a bioterrorist attack (infectious disease precautions).

15. Definitive Medical Care

Preparedness Indicator

Demonstration of effective use of all systems for recall and augmentation of hospital staff, at multiple sites and for several types of medical personnel, in periods of peak demand, through an unannounced test or use in an actual emergency (e.g., snowstorm, hurricane, etc.).

- The hospital demonstrates procedures for recall of employees and medical staff.
  - For a community that has experienced a major emergency, the hospital has activated an emergency recall plan and staff have responded.
  - The hospital has conducted an unannounced test of its recall system within the past year, and at least 80 percent of the staff whose response was requested responded within 2 hours
  - .The recall plan includes logistics and planning personnel (plant operations staff, support staff, etc.) as well as operations personnel (medical and nursing staff, etc).
- The recall plan is functionally constructed so that it can occur in a timely fashion and provides adequate information for personnel to respond adequately.

- Contact information is correct for at least four of five staff members in a test by or for site visitor.
- The hospital has established and can provide written agreements with third-party agencies for augmentation of personnel.
- All health care providers in the community have developed a coordinated plan for augmentation of personnel.
    - Minutes of a meeting showing that providers supplied information on augmentation plans and that duplications were identified and prioritized.
- The hospital's medical staff office has a list of all physicians in the community and their clinical privileges at other community hospitals.

Preparedness Indicator

Documented resolution of any issues related to cross-jurisdictional licensure and liability coverage.

- The hospital has planned for liability coverage of volunteer physicians and nurses.
    - A "Good Samaritan" law absolving physician and nurse volunteers of liability except for gross negligence protects staff.
    - The hospital's liability coverage includes a "Good Samaritan" provision.

Preparedness Indicator

Percentage of hospitals, clinics, HMOs, etc contacted in 1 hour during weekly notification checks of procedures for notification that a potential mass casualty incident has occurred.

- A log indicates that weekly notification checks are being performed.
- A log confirms that 80 percent of facilities were notified within 1 hour.

Preparedness Indicator

Time from initial notification to initiation of hospital disaster plan or incident command system.

- Evidence shows that operational incident management is in place within 20 minutes of notification.
- Evidence shows that hospital emergency operations are being

implemented at the operational level within 5 minutes of hospital notification (operational personnel are implementing their assignments).

Preparedness Indicator

Availability of all essential antidotes, antibiotics, and immune sera, in appropriate quantities, for inspection by site-visit team or peer reviewer.

- Pharmacies at two or three hospitals have sufficient ciprofloxacin or doxycycline to start treatment or prophylaxis of 100 patients and a sufficient 2-pralidoxime (2-PAM) and atropine supply for 25 patients, as well as written protocols for obtaining more ciprofloxacin, 2-PAM, and atropine quickly.
- Inventory lists include all pharmaceuticals required by the most current MMRS medical protocols.
- The pharmacists visited know the locations, contents, and procedures for accessing the local MMRS cache.
- ED staffs at two or three hospitals are able to demonstrate the protocol for securing within 24 hours 100 intensive care unit ventilators, of which at least 33 are appropriate for children.
- The response time required to make available the appropriate antidotes or antibiotics for the hypothesized number of casualties has been tested.
- Memoranda of understanding or other collaborative agreements with other local medical care facilities are available for the emergency loan and distribution of required equipment and pharmaceuticals, including pediatric ventilators.

Preparedness Indicator

Demonstration of knowledge of relevant treatment protocols by EDs, intensive care units, and primary care physicians and nurses in responses to peer-reviewer questions, exercise, or actual event.

- The medical treatment protocols for patients affected by the agents specified in the MMRS program contract (nerve agents; blister agents; choking agents; blood agents; and those responsible for anthrax, botulism, hemorrhagic fever, plague, smallpox, and tularemia) are readily located by ED staff in two or three hospitals.
- Health care professionals provide evidence of certification or other nationally recognized affirmation of CBR agent-specific knowledge and skills, if such means for certification become available in the future.
- Simulated patients presenting to two or three area EDs with signs and symptoms of smallpox are diagnosed accurately and isolated effec-

tively, appropriate staff and community officials are notified, and appropriate supportive care is arranged as needed. (Hospitals must be warned that simulated patients of some sort may be a part of the site visit.)

- For the most recent tuberculosis patient, the time from examination to the time of isolation was less than 1 hour.
- Isolation rooms are available, in the ED and other departments.
- No tuberculosis patients have been admitted to nonisolation rooms in previous 6 months.
- No staff have been furloughed due to exposure to patients with varicella, rubella, or other infectious diseases in the previous 6 months.

16. Mental Health Services for Responders, Victims, Caregivers, and Their Families

Preparedness Indicator

After-action reports from other kinds of disasters or exercises that document the coordination, availability, use, and effectiveness of mental health professionals.

Preparedness Indicator

Agreements with private organizations and individual practitioners to provide mental health services for all segments of the population.

- Evidence of practitioner training or experience providing services to disaster victims and responders is available.

Preparedness Indicator

Written procedures for provision of on-scene and community support.

17. Volunteer Utilization and Control

Preparedness Indicator

The lead voluntary agency maintains an inventory of trained volunteers for mental and physical health, family services, and other purposes.

- The agency meets the following standards for a response to terrorist events:
    - The agency recruits and trains one disaster-related mental health worker and one disaster-related physical health services worker for every 200 individuals to be affected (minimum of 250 workers).

 ◦ The agency recruits and trains up to five expert family services workers.

 ◦ The response also includes public affairs and fund-raising activities in support of service delivery as a result of a disaster.

- The agency is able to provide a list of active volunteers, how they were recently trained, and if and why they were recently activated.

Preparedness Indicator

The lead voluntary agency responds to disaster events within 2 hours of notification. This response includes shelter, feeding, disaster health services, disaster mental health services, damage assessment, and family services, as appropriate.

- After-action reports from exercises or prior disaster events are provided.
- CBR agent-related or other mass-casualty exercises are directly observed during an on-site visit.

Preparedness Indicator

"Spontaneous" volunteers are effectively screened, oriented and trained, given identification, and deployed.

- Written policies and procedures address "vetting" of volunteers and their effective incorporation into community response efforts.
- "Spontaneous" volunteers introduced into exercises and site-visit scenario-driven discussions are effectively incorporated into the community response.
- Agreements have been established with all relevant agencies on needs for and use of volunteers.

Preparedness Indicator

Demonstration that the language and the demography and culture of the communities that the volunteers serve are kept in mind when the volunteers are selected and trained.

- The agency has up-to-date language and demographic profiles of the communities that it serves and recruits and trains volunteer and paid staff to reflect those profiles.
- At the request of the site visitor, the lead agency can contact health and family services workers with locally relevant non-English-language skills.

18. Crowd and Traffic Control

Preparedness Indicator

After-action reports document crowd and traffic control at events with large attendances such as sporting events, concerts, and political conventions and prior natural or technological disasters.

- In large cities the police handle large crowds and traffic control at events on a weekly basis. These include professional sporting events (e.g., football games, which 60,000 to 80,000 people attend; baseball games, which 25,000 to 50,000 people attend; basketball and hockey games, which 10,000 to 25,000 people attend); NASCAR races, which 100,000-plus people attend; as well as festivals, parades, and conventions. If there are no significant problems at the event, after-action activities most often involve a meeting in which key participants discuss things that could be improved for the next similar event.

Preparedness Indicator

An established plan provides for crowd control at special events and during civil disturbances.

- The plan includes provisions for responsibility for incident command.
- The plan addresses coordination between government and public utilities and among the various levels of government.
- The plan includes provisions for the call-up of personnel and resource allocation.
  - Calls to a random sample show that telephone and page numbers are up to date.
  - The frequency of system tests is obtained.
  - The results of the most recent test are obtained.
- The plan provides for the handling of mass arrests.
- The plan provides for the handling of mass casualties.
- The plan includes a security plan for potential treatment facilities and their personnel, including:
  - controlled access to the facility,
  - controlled access to the grounds,
  - traffic control measures, and
  - a clear definition of hospital security and police roles and responsibilities.

Preparedness Indicator

Officers receive regular training in crowd control.

- Every officer should receive basic training in the police academy and then refresher training every 2 or 3 years. The training should cover, among other things:
    - expectations for various types of events,
    - crowd control measures,
    - understanding of the impact of deploying various chemical munitions, and
    - the use and testing of gas masks.
- Other officers should receive more specialized training at a much greater frequency.
    - Many police agencies use "field force" techniques developed in Miami and Dade County, Florida, in the 1980s following several riots. These officers should receive initial training of 2 or 3 days and then refresher training at least once a year (in Charlotte, North Carolina, about 400 officers have received this training).
    - Special Weapons and Tactics (SWAT) teams should train every month to deal with armed and barricaded subjects and high-risk entries.
    - Any specialized team that would be called out during a situation involving a CBR agent should receive training and conduct exercises on a monthly basis.
- Lesson plans, supporting procedural documents, attendance records documenting participation and proficiency, schedules for future training, and after-action reviews of exercises should all be available.

Preparedness Indicator

Adequate protective equipment is available for police officers.

- Specialized teams that would be called out during a situation involving a CBR agent and that include police should be equipped with personal protective equipment ranging from level D to level A.
- Depending on the community, one might see all officers with gas masks and helmets for use in riot control situations. Properly fitted gas masks might provide a minimal level of short-term protection against some hazards.
- Field force officers should be fully equipped with crowd control gear, in addition to gas masks and helmets.
- The "appropriate" level of protective gear for police officers not in a designated response role is difficult to establish. At a minimum, an

assessment has been made and action taken to provide whatever personal protective equipment that assessment supports.

19. Evacuation and Quarantine Decisions and Operations

Preparedness Indicator

A written plan that includes procedures for deciding upon and implementing public safety measures such as providing shelter in place, conducting an orderly evacuation, quarantining of individuals and geographical areas, and isolating patients or groups of patients.

- The plan does not need to be specific to CBR agent-related events.
- Legal authority for the decision maker is established and documented in the plan.
- Plans provide for the medical care of quarantined individuals.
- Plans provide for the nonmedical care of quarantined or isolated individuals.
- A written plan for the media includes prepared information and fact sheets explaining the need for and processes for the implementation of evacuation or quarantine.

Preparedness Indicator

Identified leadership can verbalize the contents of the procedure for the evacuation of a contaminated facility.

- The responsible entity has reviewed the experience of the state, county, and city with the evacuation of facilities that have occurred during previous emergency or urgent conditions.
- The evacuation plan has been practiced during disaster exercises (as evaluated by examination of after-action reports).

Preparedness Indicator

The identified leadership can verbalize the contents of the procedure for the initiation of isolation or quarantine.

- The responsible entity has reviewed the experience of the state, county, and city with isolations or quarantines that have occurred during previous public health operations.
- The isolation or quarantine plan has been practiced during disaster exercises (as evaluated by examination of after-action reports).

20. Fatality Management

Preparedness Indicator

Contingency contracts or other arrangements for storage capacity with local hospital morgues, mortuaries, warehouses, other facilities with cold-storage capabilities, and sources of refrigerated trucks.

Preparedness Indicator

Evidence of NDMS support and procedures for activation.

- The lead agency provides evidence of joint training or tabletop demonstration of interface with Disaster Mortuary Operational Response Teams.

Preparedness Indicator

Hands-on demonstration of decontamination can be provided in an exercise or actual incident.

- The MMRS plan identifies required decontamination equipment and the basis for the choices of particular types and quantities of equipment.
  - The equipment chosen is adequate to support the decontamination of up to 1,000 victims of a terrorist incident involving chemical agents.
- Inspection of at least one site confirms that the equipment is in inventory and is readily accessible.
  - The on-site inventory complies with the plan.
  - If the equipment is stored in a locked area, staff can locate the key without assistance.
- The necessary equipment can be set up and functioning within 30 minutes of arrival on site.
  - Procedures for expedient decontamination and keeping ambulatory victims on site for 30 minutes are in place.
  - Equipment setup is not dependent solely on members of the hazmat unit.
  - Training required for both setup and operation has been provided to enough personnel to ensure the capability of equipment operation at all times (24 hours a day, 7 days a week, every day of the year).

Preparedness Indicator

Evidence that standard operating procedures are available at morgue facilities in sufficient quantity to distribute to any expedient sites and that the required personnel are available.

21. Environmental Cleanup, Physical Restoration of Facilities, and Certification of Safety

Preparedness Indicator

Demonstration of an effective process for the identification of environmental risk and determination of the need for decontamination or vector intervention in response to questioning by the peer reviewer or by performance in an exercise, actual hazmat event, or disease outbreak.

- Review of the MMRS plan shows that it includes provisions for determination of risk and the need for decontamination or vector intervention and patient treatment.
    - The agencies and organizations required to do the following tasks have been identified:
        i. determine the existence and nature of hazardous materials or the existence and nature of vectors,
        ii. communicate findings to all MMRS response and management elements,
        iii. communicate messages to the public, and
        iv. carry out long-term surveillance and cleanup of the affected area, as required.
    - Agreements are in place to secure additional (decontamination) response elements (personnel, supplies, and equipment).
    - A training and exercise program is available to support the system and protocols.
- An on-site visit to a hazmat response team, an EMS unit, a hospital ED, or some other organization is made to observe the procedures and protocols used to identify environmental risk and determine the need for decontamination or vector intervention. A sample of personnel is able to
    - demonstrate the use of detection and agent identification equipment,
    - demonstrate the use of personal protective equipment, and
    - demonstrate use of a field management system for incorporation of specialty environmental resource agencies into the MMRS plan.

22. Follow-up Study of Responder, Caregiver, and Victim Health

Preparedness Indicator

The response plan includes a practical process for scientific investigation of human health effects in responders, caregivers, and victims.

- The local public health system has a written protocol for follow-up investigation of the human health effects (short term and long term), including the following:
  - an assessment of the nature and magnitude of the incident, including the agent(s) involved and the population affected;
  - a process for assessing the availability of resources, including the appropriate personnel, equipment, budget, treatment, and laboratory capacities;
  - baseline health data on designated emergency response personnel;
  - the identification of the "study" population and a control population, if appropriate; and
  - a communications strategy for reporting the process and results of the study to the community.

23. Process for Continuous Evaluation of Needs and Resources

Preparedness Indicator

Possession of a collection of after-action reports by all participating agencies and institutions.

- On-site indications that key agency participants have actually received after-action reports are available.
- After-action reports for exercises and major events requiring emergency management are available. They should include, at a minimum:
  - a description of the exercise or incident,
  - the objectives of the exercise,
  - the roles played by various agencies and key individuals (public and private, both inside and outside the governmental unit preparing the report),
  - a list of problems or shortcomings encountered,
  - an assessment of the reasons that these problems or shortcomings occurred, and
  - an analysis of lessons for improved future performance.

• In the absence of relevant after-action reports, written indications should assign responsibility for preparation of the reports to a particular agency or individual or should describe a procedure for assigning ad hoc responsibility in advance of planned exercises or immediately after the event for unplanned emergency management situations.

Preparedness Indicator

• During-action reports from extended exercises or prolonged responses to actual CBR agent or hazmat events
• On-site indications that key agency participants have actually received reports are available.
• Reports should include, at a minimum:
  ◦ a description of the exercise or incident,
  ◦ the objectives of the exercise,
  ◦ the roles played by various agencies and key individuals (public and private, both inside and outside the governmental unit preparing the report),
  ◦ a list of problems or shortcomings encountered,
  ◦ an assessment of the reasons that these problems or shortcomings occurred, and
  ◦ an analysis of alterations in the community response required for meeting evolving needs.
• In the absence of relevant during-action reports, written procedures should assign responsibility for preparation of the reports to a particular agency or individual or should describe a procedure for assigning ad hoc responsibility for monitoring planned exercises or unplanned emergency management situations for unanticipated developments.

Preparedness Indicator

Evidence for changes in structure or functioning in response to reported deficiencies.

• A distribution list or lists for different types of after-action reports should be available so that findings can be disseminated to participants, supervisors, and policy officials.
• A procedure for securing reviews of and comments on reports by other participants or close observers of the events covered should be in place.
  ◦ At a minimum, these should be in writing.
  ◦ For major exercises or events, provision should also be made for in-person discussions by key agency officials.

- The lead agency provides files of written comments and minutes of meetings that discuss the findings, including evidence of agreement on steps taken in light of identified problems or shortcomings.
- A procedure for generating and assigning responsibility for recommended steps to maintain or improve preparedness should be in place.
- Procedures for assigning responsibility for subsequent follow-up should be in place to see whether the proposed steps have been taken or, if not, whether the problems or shortcomings have been addressed in another appropriate way.
- Memos or meeting minutes indicating the following should also be available:
    - that subsequent follow-up of the steps has occurred and that any incomplete steps are still being monitored,
    - that substitute actions have been scheduled, or
    - that analysis of obstacles and a search for workable solutions are ongoing.

EXERCISES AND DRILLS

The committee members began their task with the common view that, in the absence of regularly occurring CBR terrorism incidents, the plans produced by MMRS program cities might be best evaluated by large-scale field exercises that would simulate such incidents and more specialized drills that would test the performances of specialized portions of the overall response plan. A proposal debated early in the committee's discussions was to design an exercise(s) that would constitute a comprehensive test of each city's response plan. The evaluation would then simply involve conducting the exercise and observing the response. This proposal was ultimately rejected as being too expensive in terms of the financial cost for OEP and in terms of time for local emergency response and medical personnel, difficult to tailor to 100 different locales, and in the case of a covert release of a biological agent, impossible to simulate realistically and ethically. Several members also observed that in their experiences it had been the planning rather than the conduct of exercises that was of greater value to the community.

One of the MMRS program contract deliverables in fact calls for a schedule of exercises, and another calls for the collection and distribution of after-action reports, so the committee opted to incorporate these exercises into the overall evaluation plan. Observers, preferably members of the team that will subsequently conduct a site visit to a community conducting an exercise, should attend large-scale exercises and significant drills before they plan a site visit. Despite the drawbacks mentioned in the previous paragraph, many of the essential capabilities can best be assessed in this fashion, and some can only be assessed in this manner. Table 8-1 and the associated preparedness criteria can serve as guides for these observers, who should be required to produce written reports of their observations and judgments of preparedness for each of the essential capabilities with an X in the column of Table 8-1 labeled "Drill." Given the expense and difficulty of planning and conducting a large scale exercise, OEP should also consider sharing these observations, suitably redacted to maintain security, with other MMRS program cities, perhaps by means of its password-limited website

SITE VISITS AND PEER EVALUATORS

Although the details of any site visit to some extent will be specific to the site being visited, the committee envisions a typical site visit consisting of a 3-day evaluation. The assessment team would gather on the afternoon or evening of Day 1 to meet, confirm assignments, and distribute the required materials. Day 2 would be devoted to individual interviews and observations, as would the morning of Day 3. Two scenario-driven group discussions would take place simultaneously on the afternoon of Day 3 (see below for more detail), and at least two assessment team members would attend each scenario. Debriefing of the team (i.e., when team members discuss their observations with each other) would take place on the morning of Day 4, and on the afternoon of Day 4, the team would debrief the community (i.e., provide some very general feedback on the team's observations and conclusions). A formal report would be produced in the ensuing month by OEP staff or their representatives and would be based on the collective observations of the assessment team.

The assessment team should consist of five individuals collectively experienced in a variety of disciplines and professions. Their task is a broad one, and it is important that they be, and be perceived as, peers of the individuals being assessed. To this end the committee recommends that the team comprise a fire department representative familiar with hazmat operations; a city- or county-level emergency manager; a local public health officer familiar with surveillance systems; an individual with extensive managerial, operational, and clinical experience in the field of prehospital emergency medical services; and an acute-care medical practitioner, who could be a nurse or a physician, with clinical experience in infectious diseases or emergency medicine and mass-casualty operations. In practice, such a team would no doubt need one or two administrative support personnel. Consideration should also be given to including OEP's regional Public Health Service emergency coordinator on the assessment team. This individual generally has served as the contracting officer's technical representative for the MMRS program contract. Inclusion on the team may produce a conflict of interest for the emergency coordinator, but he or she will also bring substantial important information regarding the local MMRS program. Similarly, the committee recommends that at least three of the five members have some previous involvement with the MMRS in their own community.

Both the community and the prospective site visitors should be notified at least six months in advance of the anticipated visit. This will allow both the community and the site visitors time to make necessary logistical arrangements, gather documents, and arrange schedules of likely participants. It will also allow OEP to gather necessary documents, review reports from previously observed exercise and drills in the community, and schedule some pre-visit training for the site visitors, which will be vital to insuring a consistent and valid assessment program.

Some pilot testing will be necessary to confirm the feasibility of this suggested approach, check interobserver reliability, and make changes where the committee's suggestions cannot be implemented. In doing this pilot testing OEP should endeavor to include communities it has some reason to believe lie at of the extremes of the preparedness continuum. It seems unlikely that all MMRS communities are equally well prepared, despite OEP intentions, and an assessment program should at least be able to distinguish the extremes of systemic or societal preparedness.

Finally, it should be obvious that the assessment program being proposed here will entail considerable expense (comparable site visits to Urban Search and Rescue Teams cost approximately $30,000 each, and OEP has already let more than 100 MMRS contracts). The program will also make substantial demands of the time of OEP staff; the committee believes this task will necessitate at least one professional position.

SCENARIO-DRIVEN GROUP INTERACTION

Every site visit will involve not only individual interviews and observations but also two simultaneous 3-hour group meetings, each facilitated by two on-site evaluators, in which a group of 12 to 15 representatives from the community's safety and health institutions will be required to answer questions about their community's response to a fictional CBR terrorism incident. The models and scenarios are adaptations of three FEMA courses designed to help senior local government officials improve their abilities to respond to mass-casualty incidents involving the use of CBR weapons (Federal Emergency Management Agency, 2001c, d, e, f). Because of the overarching importance of interagency, intergovernmental, and public-private cooperation and coordination, the goal of this portion of the site visit is to give the community a chance to demonstrate the existence of a well-understood process to coordinate all necessary capabilities to respond to a mass-casualty CBR terrorism incident, specifically, the ability to acquire, process, and appropriately distribute information required to effectively manage critical functions during an incident. The fact that the evaluators will conduct two parallel discussions will ensure that this ability is not confined to a single individual or a single individual in each institution.

Appendix F provides scenarios, discussion questions, and instructional material for the facilitators and evaluators (these roles should be assigned to different members of the site visit team). The scenarios involving chemical and radiological agents have been taken from the FEMA courses almost intact, but the FEMA scenario involving a biological agent, which involves an attack with anthrax, has been extensively modified to reflect both the knowledge about anthrax gained in the autumn of 2001 and the committee's desire to include a scenario based on a truly covert release of a biological agent. The materials from the FEMA courses are designed to support either 3-day or 1-day courses, so considerable editing of discussion questions was necessary. Much of that was accomplished by focusing on coordination and cooperation (Do the participants know each other, and how they are supposed to interact?) rather than details of individual performance (Does the city have an adequate cache of equipment and supplies? Do the physicians in the community know how to handle a suspected smallpox case?), which will be assessed in other portions of the evaluation.

The participants should be selected by the leaders of the local MMRS. The committee recommends that OEP tell the local MMRS contact only that there will be two simultaneous scenario-driven group discussions and that OEP suggest that he or she should invite representatives of all the major agencies and institutions necessary for an effective response to a mass-casualty terrorism event. In most cases it will not be possible to have all the participating jurisdictions represented, but representatives of local agencies and institutions should not all be from the same jurisdiction. OEP should ask to review the list of invitees before the site visit and should take that opportunity to suggest additions that might be crucial to the discussion. Before the site visit OEP should also attempt to identify some potential critics of the local system, with or without the aid of the local MMRS leaders, and invite them to participate as well.

SUMMARY

The survey described in the previous chapter provides one tool for assessing the effectiveness of the MMRS program, namely, a survey soliciting the opinions of the communities themselves. This chapter complements that approach by presenting the committee's recommendations for an independent and systematic assessment of the response capabilities of the large metropolitan areas that have or will participate in the MMRS program.

Several important assumptions or principles underlie these recommendations:

- Evaluation should be part of a continuous learning and continuous quality improvement program, not a one-time snapshot. This implies a continuing relationship between the communities and their evaluators that includes financial as well as technical and educational support.
- "Preparedness" is a meaningless abstract concept without a specific threat; it should be seen as a process rather than a state.
- Preparedness requires not only numerous specific capabilities, typically the responsibilities of independent offices, agencies, and institutions, but also seamless coordination of those capabilities into a coherent response. The former may be envisioned as the teeth of a comb, the latter as the base or backbone of the comb.
- Information and the ability to acquire, process, and appropriately distribute it to essential sites and personnel are central to the effective management of critical incidents including terrorism in its many forms.
- Evaluation is an exercise designed to guide distribution of local, state, and federal resources. Evaluations should be valued and understood as an opportunity for local communities to determine the areas in need of improvement and support rather than as a test of communities' self-reliance.
- A relatively small subset of the nearly 500 preparedness indicators identified in the Phase I report (Institute of Medicine, 2001) can be used to identify critical areas in need of improvement for a given community.

A set of 23 essential capabilities needed for an effective response to CBR terrorism was presented and used to guide the selection of a subset of preparedness indicators for use in a formal evaluation program. For each of those indicators, the committee then provided its opinion on what would constitute acceptable evidence of preparedness (preparedness criteria).

The chapter concludes with the committee's recommendations on methods for gathering that evidence. Evaluations by OEP should be multilevel processes that include (1) periodic review of documents and records, (2) observation of community-initiated exercises and drills, and (3) an on-site assessment. The committee views the on-site assessment as constituting both interviews with individuals about specific capabilities and a scenario-driven group interaction focused on interagency and institutional cooperation and coordination.

9

Closing Remarks

The charge to the Institute of Medicine's (IOM's) Committee on the Evaluation of the Metropolitan Medical Response System Program was to identify or develop performance measures and systems to assess the effectiveness of and identify barriers related to the Metropolitan Medical Response System (MMRS) development process and then to establish appropriate evaluation methods, tools, and processes.

Phase I of this project focused on identifying potential performance measures and systems. In Phase II, the committee used the performance measures developed in Phase I to develop appropriate evaluation methods, tools, and processes to assess the MMRS development process, both at the national level (program management) and at the local level (program success). The charge to the committee included a number of specific questions that staff of the Office of Emergency Preparedness (OEP) posed to help clarify the goals of the project. The questions associated with Phase I were answered in the Phase I report (Institute of Medicine, 2001). Those for Phase II are as follows:

a. What is the most appropriate approach or model to evaluate the MMRS development process (e.g., surveys, interviews, review of plans, peer review, operational tests, etc.)?

b. Is there an appropriate sample size from which the impact of the MMRS development process could adequately be gauged?

c. Considering the variance in local health systems, how can OEP appropriately draw meaningful conclusions from the results of this evaluation?

The primary products of this report clearly answer question (a):

- a questionnaire survey on program management, to be answered by OEP's primary point of contact in each MMRS community;
- a list of essential capabilities for effective response to chemical, biological, and radiological (CBR) terrorism, with associated preparedness indicators; and
- a three-element evaluation procedure designed to measure program success. The three elements are review of written documents and data, a site visit by a team of peer reviewers, and observations at exercises and drills and are complementary means of analyzing the community's response capabilities.

The answer to question (b), on the appropriate sample size with which the impact of the MMRS program can be gauged, is also clear, but no doubt less satisfying. As noted elsewhere in the report, in the absence of any proper control cities or pre-MMRS program data, it will be impossible to unequivocally assign credit to OEP for high states of preparedness. Most of the larger cities have received training and equipment from the U.S. Department of Defense or the U.S. Department of Justice, some have received grants and training from the Centers for Disease Control and Prevention, and all have spent time and money from state and local budgets. The MMRS program's emphasis on multiagency, multijurisdictional planning has undoubtedly played a major role in increasing preparedness in many cities, but no large city could become well prepared solely as a result of the relatively meager funding provided by the OEP contracts. Technically, then, there is no sample size that will allow valid generalization about the impact of the MMRS program.

Given this answer to question (b), the answer to question (c) on just what conclusions OEP can draw from the use of the committee's suggested evaluation tools becomes very important, and it is embodied in what were called "guiding principles" in Chapter 8. The first of these was that the committee believes that program assessment is primarily for the purpose of identifying and correcting shortfalls in OEP's MMRS program. At the community level, evaluation is an exercise designed to guide the distribution of local, state, and federal resources. This evaluation should be valued and understood as an opportunity for local communities to determine the areas in need of improvement and support rather than as a test of communities' self-reliance. In fact, the committee believes that few if any communities would receive high grades on all essential capabilities if the recommended evaluation program began tomorrow.

A second and equally important principle holds that evaluation should be part of a continuous learning and continuous quality improvement program, not a one-time snapshot. That is, readiness should be seen as a process rather than a state. This implies a continuing relationship between the communities and their evaluators that includes financial as well as technical and educational support. When this study began in the autumn of 2000, the notion of a continuing financial relationship with even a small subset of MMRS program cities would have seemed pointless, given the limited OEP budget and the mandate to develop programs in the 120 largest cities. As this report is being written in April 2002, however, the U.S. Department of Health and Human Services (DHHS) had begun distributing funds from the more than $2.9 billion of fiscal year (FY) 2002 supplemental appropriations to address bioterrorism. That is almost 10 times the amount available in FY 2001. More than $1 billion of that total is designated to help states prepare their public health infrastructures to respond to a bioterrorism attack (U.S. Department of Health and Human Services, 2002). The $51 million allocated to OEP for support of community emergency preparedness includes funding for an additional 25 cities, which, according to DHHS, means that 80 percent of the U.S. population is covered by an MMRS plan. Also included in DHHS spending plans for FY 2002 is $518 million to enhance preparedness at the nation's hospitals, which, as the committee has already noted (Institute of Medicine, 2001), have been particularly difficult to incorporate into MMRS programs.

Given these caveats, how can OEP best use the data from the proposed evaluation program?

STRATEGIC USES OF EVALUATION DATA: IMPLEMENTING THE "LAYERING STRATEGY"

Chapter 5 outlined a variety of evaluation functions and addressed the issue of how these might be combined through various kinds of data collection and analysis. This "layering strategy" optimizes the use of these data at a reasonable cost.

The strategy relies on several assumptions. First, it assumes that the funded cities will indeed provide valid information in the spirit of continuous quality improvement. Particularly in the wake of the events of September 11, 2001, emergency managers and other personnel of major cities have been subject to criticism that is not conducive to problem solving. Chapter 5 outlined the problem of "corruptibility of indicators": if blame accrues to the assessment of preparedness, the data cannot be valid and problems are unlikely to be addressed. As the committee has indicated, there is no such thing as perfect preparedness.

The second assumption is that a variety of stakeholders at the federal, state, and local levels will continue to pose questions about preparedness that require different levels of data aggregation. Not all these questions can be anticipated, so OEP may wish to have a portfolio of findings prepared in advance. To understand the needs of stakeholders, especially the policy makers, it is best to engage them when data collection is being planned. This cannot be done when decisions are imminent; it requires substantial lead time (Leviton and Boruch, 1984). Later in this chapter the committee provides some suggestions on how to do this.

The third assumption is that even with more abundant resources, not all preparedness indicators can be monitored equally well, all the time, in all metropolitan areas. Therefore, OEP will need to be judicious about the questions that it addresses and the breadth and depth with which it addresses those questions. The trade-offs between data collection for intensity, validity, and discovery versus data collection for breadth and prevalence have been amply described in the evaluation literature, as have methods that can be used to balance the two to optimize the utility of the information obtained (Cronbach, 1982). However, there are several ways to leverage a bigger return on investment in data collection. One of them is the "evaluation funnel."

As outlined in previous chapters, the backbone of evaluation for any MMRS is the peer-review site visit. The site visits will provide more valid and intensive data than documents, reports, surveys, and other methods used to obtain a breadth of data. The site visits are important to provide the formative feedback and to let OEP know about the levels of preparedness in individual metropolitan areas. However, site visits are expensive and time-consuming, and by themselves they cannot give OEP the summative data it requires to assess overall MMRS program performance and identify chronic areas in need of improvement across metropolitan areas.

To address this problem, evaluation in other policy areas has adopted an approach best described as an "evaluation funnel." The evaluation funnel approach permits evaluators to first obtain a large amount of imprecise information; the evaluators then focus on the collection of more in-depth data. The evaluation funnel idea would work as follows for the MMRS program: (1) a large amount of basic information would be obtained on all program sites, (2) the evaluators would confer with program stakeholders to identify dimensions of interest for further study, and (3) the evaluators would collect more in-depth data for a sample of sites. These three stages of the evaluation funnel approach are described in more detail below.

1. Basic information on program sites. In the case of the MMRS program, data collection for the first stage of the evaluation funnel approach would consist of the cross-tabulation of data and information from the final reports (plans) of the MMRS program communities by gathering

periodic reports with very specific templates for information (the written indicators in Table 8-1) or by surveying lead agencies across sites on a periodic basis (the contractor survey described in Chapter 7). This stage can be broad but shallow, in the sense that one does not obtain data and information beyond those available in the documentation or seek to establish the validity of self-reports. The products of this stage include an overview of a program's status that can later be validated by sampling, a sense of the most pressing self-reported chronic problems across the MMRS program communities, and an overview of program characteristics and activities and the most important variations among programs.

2. Identify dimensions of interest for further study. The purpose of this stage of the evaluation funnel approach is to understand the most important characteristics of the MMRS program and how they vary among the MMRS program communities to prepare for the later collection of more in-depth data. At this point, OEP would want to present the results of Stage 1 of its evaluation to the key stakeholders for comment. What was revealing to them? What was of concern? What are the most important components or elements about the different MMRS programs to be studied in depth later? The importance of this consultation step cannot be overstated. It is a key element to ensuring relevant and useful evaluations and can also guide sampling strategies for more intensive data collection (during site visits). The products of Stage 2 include input so that OEP can anticipate questions that stakeholders (such as the U.S. Congress) are likely to pose later and a sampling frame that can be used to choose MMRS program communities for further in-depth investigation through site visits.

3. In-depth study of a sample of MMRS program communities. The site visits conducted by peers described in Chapter 8 would be used to study samples of the MMRS program communities. If a large number of site visits can be budgeted, a formal sampling frame becomes feasible, based on deliberations conducted during Stage 2. When it is not possible to sample a sufficient number of MMRS program sites to achieve statistically significant differences, dimensions of particular interest can be chosen. In this way, the evaluators would be able to evaluate sites that achieve the mode for a particular dimension as well as several sites that vary from the mode in a particular dimension. For example, even before consultation with stakeholders, it might be anticipated that the number of jurisdictions involved is likely to be a dimension of interest. OEP might sample one or more metropolitan areas with the average number of jurisdictions in an MMRS program and then deliberately include MMRS program communities that involve far more or far fewer jurisdictions than the mode. The choice of criteria for sampling sites in any given year will come from the stakeholder consultations obtained during Stage 2. The products of

the third stage can include technical assistance and formative information for individual MMRS program communities, summative evaluations of the MMRS program communities visited, validation of the self-reported information from Stage 1 (which increases confidence in the data collected during Stage 1), and finally, qualitative case study reports to stimulate discussion at both the community and the national levels. These in-depth case studies are chosen during Stage 2 to maximize relevance to policy and program needs for information.

COMMITTEE CRITIQUE AND SUGGESTIONS FOR PROGRAM AMENDMENTS

The Phase I report suggests several activities or areas that might be useful additions to future MMRS program contracts with additional cities (Institute of Medicine, 2001). Among these are a preliminary assessment of the community's strengths and weaknesses and provisions for the use and management of volunteers, for the receipt and distribution of materials from the National Pharmaceutical Stockpile, for decision making related to evacuation and disease containment, for the provision of shelters for people fleeing an area of real or perceived contamination, for postevent follow-up on the health of responders and caregivers, and for postevent amelioration of anxiety in the community at large. The preparedness indicators provided in this report should also enable OEP to operationally define the "operational capability" it demands as the capstone of its contracts. Despite these shortfalls, the committee has been favorably impressed by the MMRS program's focus on empowering local communities, as opposed to creating yet another federal team to rush to a community at the time of an incident, and the program's flexibility in allowing each community to shape its system to its unique circumstances and requirements. A carefully done evaluation program of the sort described in this report should make the MMRS program even better.

Not only does it seem that resources are now available for the continuing financial relationship suggested by the committee, but it also seems that a consensus now exists on the need for shared responsibility among a wide variety of governmental and nongovernmental agencies to achieve the goals of the MMRS program. When the committee began this project, the future success of the MMRS program depended on voluntary cooperative efforts to prepare for possible but seemingly improbable events. As the project concludes, the committee believes that OEP must be empowered to take a stance that fosters voluntary collaboration but must be willing and able to enforce integration of local, state, and federal services as a pressing societal need for coping with inevitable future acts of terrorism.

The importance of the MMRS program effort is no longer equivocal, questionable, or debatable. The philosophy that it has developed has become an essential and rational approach that can be truly successful only with a rigorous and continuing evaluation and improvement program. The enhanced organization and cooperation demanded by a well-functioning MMRS program will permit a unified preparedness and public health system with immense potential for improved responses not only to a wide spectrum of terrorist acts but also to mass-casualty incidents of all varieties.

References

Advisory Panel to Assess Domestic Response Capabilities for Terrorism Involving Weapons of Mass Destruction. 2000. *Second Annual Report to The President and The Congress: II. Toward a National Strategy for Combating Terrorism.* Washington, DC: RAND.

Baessler CA. 2000. Are educational interventions enough for retention of cardiopulmonary resuscitation techniques? *Critical Care Medicine* 28(9):3363–3364.

Beauchesne A. 2001. *Natural Disasters: A Governor's Guide to Emergency Management,* Vol. 1. Washington, DC: National Governor's Association. [Online]. Available: http://www.nga.org/cda/files/REPORTEMERGUIDE2001.pdf [accessed February 18, 2002].

Blau, PM. 1963. *The Dynamics of Bureaucracy,* 2nd edition. Chicago: University of Chicago Press.

Broomfield R. 1996. A quasi-experimental research to investigate the retention of basic cardiopulmonary resuscitation skills and knowledge by qualified nurses following a course in professional development. *Journal of Advanced Nursing* 23(5):1016–1023.

Bush, GW. 2001. Executive Order Establishing the Office of Homeland Security and the Homeland Security Council [Online]. Available: http://www.whitehouse.gov/news/releases/2001/10/20011008-2.html [accessed October 8, 2001]

California Office of Emergency Services. 2002. *Governor's Office of Emergency Services Origins and Development: A Chronology 1917-1999.* [Online]. Available: http://www.oes.ca.gov [accessed February 18, 2002] .

Campbell DT. 1988. *Methodology and Epistemology for Social Science: Selected Papers.* Chicago: University of Chicago Press.

Centers for Disease Control and Prevention. 2001a. Update: investigation of bioterrorism-related anthrax and interim guidelines for exposure management and antimicrobial therapy, October 2001. *Morbidity and Mortality Weekly Report* 50(42):909–919.

Centers for Disease Control and Prevention. 2001b. Vaccinia (smallpox) vaccine recommendations of the Advisory Committee on Immunization Practices (ACIP), 2001. *Morbidity and Mortality Weekly Report* 50(RR10):1–25.

Cilluffo F, Collins JJ, de Borchgrave A, Goure D, Horowitz M. 2000. *Defending America in the 21st Century: New Challenges, New Organizations, and New Policies: Executive Summary of Four CSIS Working Group Reports on Homeland Defense*. Washington, DC: Center for Strategic and International Studies.

Cronbach LJ. 1982. *Designing Evaluations of Educational and Social Programs*. San Francisco, CA: Jossey-Bass.

Cronbach LJ, Ambron SR, Dornbusch SM, Hess RD, Hornik RC, Phillips DC,Walker DF, Weiner SS. 1980. *Toward Reform of Program Evaluation*. San Francisco, CA: Jossey-Bass.

Danon YL, Shemer J. 1994. *Chemical Warfare Medicine*. Jerusalem, Israel: Gefen.

DeMers E. 2001. *EMAP, the Emergency Management Accreditation Program*. Paper presented to the Institute of Medicine Committee on Evaluation of the Metropolitan Medical Response System Program, October 23, 2001, Washington, DC.

Disaster and Emergency Reference Center. 1998. Nimpuno K, ed. *Disaster Management Glossary*. Delft, the Netherlands: Disaster and Emergency Reference Center.

Drabek T. 1996. *The Sociology of Disasters, Instructor's Guide*. Emmitsburg, MD: Emergency Management Institute, Federal Emergency Management Agency. [Online]. Available: http://www.fema.gov/emi/edu/aem_courses.htm [accessed February 18, 2002].

Emergency Management Assistance Compact. 2002. *EMAC At-A-Glance*. [Online]. Available: http://www.nemaweb.org/EMAC/About_EMAC/What_is_Emac.cfm [accessed February 18, 2002].

Environmental Protection Agency. 1999. *NCP Overview*. [Online]. Available: http://www.epa.gov/oilspill/ncpover.htm [accessed February 18, 2002].

Federal Bureau of Investigation (2000). *Press Release on Graduation of the Final Class Taking the Weapons of Mass Destruction (WMD) Bomb Technicians Emergency Action Course*, June 29, 2000. [Online]. Available: http://www.fbi.gov/pressrel/pressrel00/wmd.htm [Accessed February 12, 2002].

Federal Emergency Management Agency. 1992. *Federal Response Plan*. [Online]. Available: http://www.fema.gov/r-n-r/frp/ [accessed December 16, 1999].

Federal Emergency Management Agency. 1995. *Introduction to Emergency Management*. Emmitsburg, MD: Emergency Management Institute.

Federal Emergency Management Agency. 1996a. *Mitigation: Minimizing the Effects of Disaster* [Online]. Available: http://www.fema.gov/mit/mitigatf.htm [accessed February 18, 2002].

Federal Emergency Management Agency. 1996b. *Guide for All-Hazard Emergency Operations Planning: State and Local Guide (101)*. [Online]. Available: http://www.fema.gov/library/allhzpln.htm [accessed April 15, 2001].

Federal Emergency Management Agency. 1997a. *Report to Congress on Response to Threats of Terrorist Use of Weapons of Mass Destruction*. Washington, DC: Federal Emergency Management Agency

Federal Emergency Management Agency. 1997b. *Multi Hazard Identification and Risk Assessment*. [Online]. Available: http://www.fema.gov/mit/tsd/dl_mhira.htm [accessed February 18, 2002].

Federal Emergency Management Agency. 1999a. *The Robert T. Stafford Disaster Relief and Emergency Assistance Act, as Amended, 42 U.S.C. 5121, et seq.* [Online]. Available: http://www.fema.gov/r-n-r/pa/pa009.htm [accessed February 18, 2002].

Federal Emergency Management Agency. 1999b. *Federal Response Plan Terrorism Incident Annex* [Online]. Available: http://www.fema.gov/r-n-r/frp/frpterr.htm [accessed February 18, 2002].

Federal Emergency Management Agency. 1999c. *Statement of Catherine H. Light, Director, Office of National Security Affairs, before the Subcommittee on Oversight, Investigations and Emergency Management of the U.S. House Committee on Transportation and Infrastructure, June 9, 1999.* [Online]. Available: http://www.fema.gov/library/light609.htm [accessed October 11, 2000].

Federal Emergency Management Agency. 2000a. *State Capability Assessment for Readiness: A Report to the United States Senate Committee on Appropriations.* Washington, DC: Federal Emergency Management Agency.

Federal Emergency Management Agency. 2000b. *Hazards, Disasters and the U.S. Emergency Management System: An Introduction: Terms and Definitions Appendix (Working draft: January 10, 2000).* [Online]. Available: http://www.fema.gov/emi/edu/hazdisusems.htm [accessed February 18, 2002].

Federal Emergency Management Agency. 2000c. *REP: Radiological Emergency Preparedness Program.* [Online]. Available: http://www.fema.gov/pte/rep/ [accessed December 16, 2000].

Federal Emergency Management Agency. 2001a. *Hazardous Materials Exercise Evaluation Supplement* [Online]. Available: http://fema.gov/pte/carep.htm [accessed April 15, 2001].

Federal Emergency Management Agency. 2001b. *CHER-CAP: Comprehensive Hazardous Materials Emergency Response Capability Assessment Program.* [Online]. Available: http://www.fema.gov/library/cher_capf.htm [accessed February 8, 2001].

Federal Emergency Management Agency. 2001c. *Terrorism Consequence Management G310—Weapons of Mass Destruction Courses and Materials.* [Online]. Available: http://www.fema.gov/emi/g310wmd.htm [accessed April 15, 2001].

Federal Emergency Management Agency. 2001d. *Weapons of Mass Destruction: Biological-Anthrax Scenario: Instructor Guide: Orientation and Exercise Course G 310.05.* [Online]. Available: ftp://ftp.fema.gov/emi/G310_05/IG/complete.pdf [accessed April 15, 2001].

Federal Emergency Management Agency. 2001e. *Weapons of Mass Destruction: Chemical-Sarin Scenario: Instructor Guide: Orientation and Exercise Course G 310.03.* [Online]. Available: ftp://ftp.fema.gov/emi/G310_03/IG/complete.pdf [accessed April 15, 2001].

Federal Emergency Management Agency. 2001f. *Weapons of Mass Destruction: Radiological Scenario: Instructor Guide: Orientation and Exercise Course G 310.02.* [Online]. Available: ftp://ftp.fema.gov/emi/G310_02/IG/complete.pdf [accessed April 15, 2001].

Federal Emergency Management Agency. 2001h. *What is CSEPP?* [Online]. Available: http://www.fema.gov/pte/csepp1.htm [accessed April 15, 2001].

Federal Emergency Management Agency. 2002a. *The Emergency Program Manager.* [Online]. Available: http://training.fema.gov/EMIWeb/crslist.htm [accessed February 18, 2002].

Federal Emergency Management Agency. 2002b. *A Guide to the Disaster Declaration Process.* Available: http://www.fema.gov/r-n-r/dec_guid.htm [accessed February 18, 2002].

Federal Emergency Management Agency. 2002c. *Federal Radiological Emergency Response Plan: Operational Plan.* [Online]. Available: http://www.au.af.mil/au/awc/awcgate/frerp/frerp.htm [accessed February 18, 2002].

Federal Emergency Management Agency and National Emergency Management Association. (1997). *State Capability Assessment for Readiness (CAR).* Washington, DC: Federal Emergency Management Agency and National Emergency Management Association.

Feldman RHL. 1985. Promoting occupational safety and health. In: Everly GS, Feldman RHK, eds. *Occupational Health Promotion: Health Behavior in the Workplace.* New York, NY: Wiley.

Fine A, Layton M. 2001. Lessons from the West Nile viral encephalitis outbreak in New York City, 1999: implications for bioterrorism preparedness. *Clinical Infectious Diseases* 32:277–282.

Francisco VT, Buterfoss FD, Capwell EM. 2001. Key issues in evaluation: quantitative and qualitative methods and research design. *Health Promotion Practice* 2(1):20-23.

Franz DR, Jahrling PB, Friedlander AM, McClain DJ, Hoover DL, Bryne WR, Pavlin JA, Christopher GW, Eitzen EM. 1997. Clinical recognition and management of patients exposed to biological warfare agents. *Journal of the American Medical Association* 278(5):399–411.

Gofrit ON, Leibovici D, Shemer J, Henig A, Shapira SC. 1997. The efficacy of integrating "smart simulated casualties" in hospital disaster plans. *Prehospital and Disaster Medicine* 12(2):97-101.

Institute of Medicine. 1999. *Chemical and Biological Terrorism: Research and Development to Improve Civilian Medical Response*. Washington, DC: National Academy Press. [Online]. Available: http://www.nap.edu/catalog/6364.html [accessed February 18, 2002].

Institute of Medicine. 2001. *Tools for Evaluating the Metropolitan Medical Response Program: Phase I Report*. Washington, DC: National Academy Press. [Online]. Available: http://www.nap.edu/catalog/10221.html [accessed February 18, 2002].

Kiehl S, Niedowski E. 2001, July 19. Battling the unknown; dangers: the chemical fire presented unusual dangers for firefighters who, with limited oxygen supplies, were unsure of what they would face; fire in the Howard Street Tunnel. *The Baltimore Sun* p. 1A.

Komaki J, Barwick KD, Scott LR. 1978. A behavioral approach to occupational safety: pinpointing and reinforcing safe performance in a food manufacturing plant. *Journal of Applied Psychology* 63:434–445.

Layton L, Phillips D. 2001, July 19. Train sets tunnel afire, shuts down Baltimore. *The Washington Post*. p. A01.

Leviton LC. 1987. Changes in Law as Leverage Points for Policy Research. *American Behavioral Scientist* 30(6) 632-643.

Leviton, LC, Boruch RF. 1983. Contributions of evaluation to education programs and policy. *Evaluation Review* 7:563–598.

Leviton LC, Boruch RF. 1984. Why the compensatory education evaluation was useful. *Journal of Policy Analysis and Management*, 3:299–305.

Lillibridge, S. 2001. CDC support to state and local programs to combat bioterrorism. Paper presented to the Institute of Medicine Committee on Evaluation of the Metropolitan Medical Response System Program, February 13, 2001, Washington, DC.

Mallonee S, Shariat S, Stennies G, Waxweiler R, Hogan D, Jordan F. 1996. Physical injuries and fatalities resulting from the Oklahoma City bombing. *Journal of the American Medical Association* 276(5):382–387.

Marrs G. 1995. Report from Fire Chief. *Fire Engineering* , 148(10). [Online]. Available: http://fe.pennnet.com/home.cfm [accessed February 16, 2002]

Maryland Emergency Management Agency. 2002. *MEMA Fact Sheet*. [Online]. Available: http://www.mema.state.md.us/about_fact.html [accessed February 18, 2002].

Nash D, Mostashari F, Fine A, Miller J, O'Leary D, Murray K, Huang A, Rosenberg A, Greenberg A, Sherman M, Wong S, Layton M. 2001. The outbreak of West Nile virus infection in the New York City area in 1999. *New England Journal of Medicine* 344(24), 1807-1814.

National Academy of Public Administration. 1993. *Coping with Catastrophe: Building an Emergency Management System to Meet People's Needs in Natural and Manmade Disasters*. Washington, DC: National Academy of Public Administration.

National Domestic Preparedness Office. 2002. *Blueprint for the National Domestic Preparedness Office.* [Online]. Available: http://www.ndpo.gov/blueprint.pdf [accessed February 12, 2002].

National Emergency Management Association. 2001. *Emergency Management Accreditation Program.* [Online]. Available: http://www.emaponline.org/index.cfm [accessed July 6, 2001].

Office of Management and Budget. 2001. *Annual Report to Congress on Combating Terrorism.* Washington, DC: Office of Management and Budget.

Rudman WB. 2001. *Prepared Statement of the Honorable Warren B. Rudman before the Subcommittee on National Security, Veterans Affairs, and International Relations of the Committee on Government Reform, U.S. House of Representatives.* Washington, DC: U.S. Commission on National Security/21st Century.

Samways MC. 1983. Cost-effective occupational health and safety training. *American Industrial Hygiene Association Journal* 44:A-6-A-9.

Scriven M. 1991. *Evaluation Thesaurus*, 4th ed. Newbury Park, CA: Sage.

Shadish WR, Cook TD, Campbell DT. 2001. *Experimental and Quasi-Experimental Designs for Generalized Causal Inference.* Boston, MA: Houghton Mifflin.

Sharp D. 2002. Can cities prepare for terrorism? Perspective from the United Kingdom. *Journal of Urban Health* 79(1):10-11.

Sidell FR, Takefuji ET, Franz DR. 1997. *Medical Aspects of Chemical and Biological Warfare.* Washington, DC: Office of the Surgeon General at TMM Publications.

Sylves R. 1998. *The Political and Policy Basis of Emergency Management, Emergency Management Institute Instructor Guide.* [Online]. Available: http://www.fema.gov/emi/edu/aem_courses.htm [accessed February 18, 2002].

Terry D. 1995, October 4. Agents in Chicago track a subtle health hazard: heat. *The New York Times.* p. A9.

U.S. Department of Health and Human Services. 1996. *Health and Medical Services Support Plan for the Federal Response to Acts of Chemical/Biological (C/B) Terrorism.* [Online]. Available: http://ndms.dhhs.gov/CT_Program/Response_Planning/C-BHMPlan.pdf [accessed January 10, 2001].

U.S. Department of Health and Human Services. 2002. *Bioterror Funding Provides Blueprint to Build a Strong New Public Health Infrastructure. HHS Fact Sheet, January 25, 2002.* [Online]. Available: http://www.hhs.gov/news/press/2002pres/20020125.html [accessed January 30, 2002].

U.S. Department of Justice. 2002a. *Office of Domestic Preparedness Equipment Acquisition Grants* [Online]. Available: http://www.ojp.usdoj.gov/odp/grants/goals.htm [accessed February 12, 2002].

U.S. Department of Justice. 2002b. *Office of Domestic Preparedness Training* [Online]. Available: http://www.ojp.usdoj.gov/odp/ta/training.htm [accessed February 12, 2002].

U.S. Department of Justice. 2002c. *Office of Domestic Preparedness Assessments* [Online]. Available: http://www.ojp.usdoj.gov/odp/assessments/definition.htm [accessed February 12, 2002].

U.S. Department of Justice. 2002d. *Office of Domestic Preparedness Exercise Development and Support* [Online]. Available: http://www.ojp.usdoj.gov/odp/ta/training.htm [accessed February 12, 2002].

U.S. Department of Justice. 2002e. *Office of Domestic Preparedness Weapons of Mass Destruction Training Program* [Online]. Available: http://www.ojp.usdoj.gov/odp/docs/coursecatalog.pdf [accessed February 12, 2002].

U.S. General Accounting Office. 2000a. *West Nile Virus Outbreak: Lessons for Public Health Preparedness.* HEHS-00-180. Washington, DC: U.S. General Accounting Office.

U.S. General Accounting Office. 2000b. *Combating Terrorism: Federal Response Teams Provide Varied Capabilities; Opportunities Remain to Improve Coordination.* GAO-01-14). Washington, DC: U.S. General Accounting Office.

U.S. General Accounting Office. 2001a. *Combating Terrorism: Selected Challenges and Related Recommendations.* GAO-01-822. Washington, DC: U.S. General Accounting Office.

U.S. General Accounting Office. 2001b. *Bioterrorism: Coordination and Preparedness.* Testimony of Janet Heinrich before the Subcommittee on Government Efficiency, Financial Management, and Intergovernmental Relations, Committee on Government Reform, U.S. House of Representatives, October 5, 2001. Report Number GAO-01-822. Washington, DC: U.S. General Accounting Office.

U.S. House of Representatives. 1998a. Departments of Commerce, Justice, and State, The Judiciary, and Related Agencies Appropriations Bill, Fiscal Year 1999. House Report 105-636. Washington, DC: U.S. House of Representatives.

U.S. House of Representatives. 1998b. Making Omnibus Consolidated and Emergency Supplemental Appropriations For Fiscal Year 1999. House Report 105-825. Washington, DC: U.S. House of Representatives.

U.S. Senate. 1998. An Original Bill Making Appropriations for the Departments of Commerce, Justice, and State, the Judiciary, and Related Agencies for the Fiscal Year Ending September 30, 1999, and for Other Purposes. Senate Report 105-235. Washington, DC: U.S. Senate.

Verger P, Aurengo A, Geoffroy B, LeGuen B. 2001. Iodine kinetics and effectiveness of stable iodine prophylaxis after intake of radioactive iodine: a review. *Thyroid* 11(4):353–360.

Zanzonico PB, Becker DV. 2000. Effects of time of administration and dietary iodine levels on potassium iodide (KI) blockade of thyroid irradiation by I-131 from radioactive fallout. *Health Physics* 78(6):660–667.

A

Committee and Staff Biographies

COMMITTEE

LEWIS GOLDFRANK, M.D. (Chair), is Director of Emergency Medicine, New York University Hospital Center, Bellevue Medical Center. He is also the medical director of the New York City Poison Control Center. Dr. Goldfrank served as president of the Society of Academic Emergency Medicine and chaired the American Board of Emergency Medicine's Subboard on Medical Toxicology. He is coeditor of the Agency for Toxic Substances Disease Registry's *Medical Guidelines for Managing Hazmat Incidents* and senior editor of *Goldfrank's Toxicologic Emergencies*, a standard text in medical toxicology. Dr. Goldfrank is a member of the Institute of Medicine and previously served on the Committee on Research and Development Needs for Improving Civilian Medical Response to Chemical and Biological Terrorism Incidents.

JOSEPH BARBERA, M.D., is Co-Director of the George Washington University Institute for Crisis, Disaster, and Risk Management. He is an Associate Professor of Engineering and Clinical Associate Professor of Emergency Medicine at The George Washington University. Dr. Barbera is residency trained in emergency medicine and family medicine and has been involved in responses to hurricanes, the Oklahoma City bombing, mine disasters, earthquakes, and biological terrorism threats since 1986. Dr. Barbera has been the lead medical consultant for the Federal Emergency Management Agency in the development of the National Urban Search & Rescue Response System and has provided extensive consultation to the U.S. Public Health Service and the U.S. Department of Veterans Affairs in the development of the National Disaster Medical System. As chair of the emergency preparedness committee for the George Washington University Hospital, Dr. Barbera oversaw implementation of a mass patient decontamination and treatment facility and worked with other hospitals to develop a similar capability for response to chemical terrorism. As founder and chair of the District of Columbia Hospital Association's Emergency Preparedness Committee, Dr. Barbera led the implementation of a comprehensive Hospital Mutual Aid System for Washington, D.C., and has been instrumental in regional emergency planning and in coordinating disaster response exercises, including the medical participation in the federal Domestic Preparedness Program's regional chemical and biological terrorism exercises. Dr. Barbera is a medical officer for the Office of Foreign Disaster Assistance International Search & Rescue Program and also provides emergency management and medical preparedness consultation to the U.S. Capitol's Office of the Attending Physician, including contingency planning for the presidential inauguration and state of the union addresses. He has provided emergency management expertise to multiple other organizations, including the White House medical staff, Walter Reed Army Medical Center, and the Washington D.C. Veterans Affairs Medical Center.

GEORGES C. BENJAMIN, M.D., was appointed secretary of Health and Mental Hygiene by Maryland Gov. Parris N. Glendening, effective May 1, 1999. He oversees an agency with more than 10,000 employees and a $4.2 billion budget. Dr. Benjamin is a graduate of the Illinois Institute of Technology and the University of Illinois College of Medicine. He is board certified in internal medicine and is a fellow of the American College of Physicians. His previous career experience includes serving in administrative positions as chief of the Acute Illness Clinic at Madigan Army Medical Center, chief of Emergency Medicine at Walter Reed Army Medical Center, chairman of the Department of Community Health and Ambulatory Care at the District of Columbia General Hospital, and health commissioner for the District of Columbia. Dr. Benjamin leads the state's public health efforts to combat biological and chemical terrorism and was a member of the Institute of Medicine's Committee on Research and Development Needs for Improving Civilian Medical Response to Chemical and Biological Terrorism Incidents.

JAMES BENTLEY, Ph.D., joined the American Hospital Association (AHA) in 1991 and is the Senior Vice President for Strategic Policy Planning at the AHA. He earned a B.A. in health facilities management from Michigan State University and a Ph.D. in medical care organization from the University of Michigan. Dr. Bentley's current responsibilities include developing AHA policy on long-term public issues, leading AHA's initiatives on workforce supply, and financing and accreditation of graduate and continuing medical education. Before joining AHA, Dr. Bentley spent 15 years with the Association of American Medical Colleges (AAMC). Initially responsible for legislative and regulatory activities affecting teaching hospitals, he concluded his AAMC career as Vice President of Clinical Services with responsibility for the association's program of services for teaching hospitals and faculty practice plans. Dr. Bentley spent 5 years in the U.S. Navy Medical Service Corps and has been on the faculty of George Washington University, where he taught medical sociology and health care administration. In 1998 and 1999, Dr. Bentley was a member of the Board of Examiners for the Malcom Baldridge National Quality Award. He has served two terms as a member of the Board of Trustees of Holy Cross Health of Silver Spring, Maryland, and continues to serve on its Mission and Planning Committee.

KENNETH I. BERNS, M.D., Ph.D. is President and Chief Executive Officer of Mount Sinai Medical Center. He is also a professor in the Departments of Microbiology and Gene Therapy. Dr. Berns completed his undergraduate requirements for biochemical sciences at Harvard University and received an A.B. with general honors in biology from Johns Hopkins University. He also earned a Ph.D. and an M.D. at Johns Hopkins University and completed his internship in pediatrics at Harriet Lane Service, Johns Hopkins Hospital. He has pioneered research on the mechanism of viral replication and has been a major contributor to understanding of the molecular mechanisms underlying replication of single-stranded viral DNA, the integration of viral DNA into the host-cell genome, and viral latency. Dr. Berns has served as co-chair for the American Society for Microbiology's Task Force on Bioterrorism, as well as for the Institute of Medicine's Resource Sharing Committee. Dr. Berns is a member of both the Institute of Medicine and the National Academy of Sciences.

RAYMOND M. DOWNEY (November 2000 to September 2001) was Chief of Rescue Operations in the New York City Fire Department's Special Operations Command, where he was responsible for preparedness, training, and response to weapons of mass destruction incidents for the department until his death in the World Trade Center attack of September 11, 2001. The command, which includes 450 firefighters and officers in 25 special units, has fully equipped and trained 12 units to respond to such incidents. Chief Downey was a member of the Advisory Panel to Assess Domestic Response Capabilities for Terrorism Involving Weapons of Mass Destruction, also known as The Gilmore Commission. Mr. Downey lectured nationally and internationally on terrorism and was one of the lead instructors at the First Worldwide Conference on Strengthening the Fire and Emergency Response to Terrorism. In addition to operating at the World Trade Center bombing in 1993, his disaster response experience included 16 days as the operations chief for the Federal Emergency Management Agency (FEMA) at the Oklahoma City bombing, the Humberto Vidal gas explosion in Puerto Rico, and numerous other hurricanes, ice storms, and floods. Mr. Downey was the task force leaders' representative to FEMA for all 28 Urban Search and Rescue teams in the National Response System, a member of FEMA's Advisory Committee for Urban Search and Rescue, and author of the book *The Rescue Company*, published by Fire Engineering Books and Videos.

FRANCES EDWARDS-WINSLOW, Ph.D., is the Director of the Office of Emergency Services for the City of San Jose, California, as well as the director of the San Jose Metropolitan Medical Task Force. Before assuming these positions, she served as Commissioner for the State of California Seismic Safety Commission. Dr. Edwards-Winslow received both a B.A. and an M.A. from Drew University. She later earned both a master of urban planning degree and a Ph.D. from New York University and a certificate in hazardous materials management from the University of California, Irvine. Dr. Winslow is a certified emergency manager and an instructor for the Federal Emergency Management Agency. She is also a member of the Stanford University Bio/Chem Warfare Working Group and a scholar for the Executive Session on Terrorism at Harvard University's Kennedy School of Government. Dr. Edwards-Winslow is affiliated with the American Society for Public Administration, for which she has served on several committees including the National Policy Issues Committee and the Section on Emergency Management.

LINDA F. FAIN served as the Disaster Assistance Coordinator for the California Department of Mental Health from 1987 until her retirement in October 2000. She developed and maintained the mental health section of the California emergency plan, provided training and technical assistance to local mental health departments, and designed and participated in federal, state, and local emergency exercises. A member of the faculty for Crisis Counseling Assistance workshops at the National Emergency Training Center and the Federal Emergency Management Agency (FEMA) Crisis Counseling Program Workgroup, she coordinated statewide response and recovery activities following 19 presidentially declared disasters, from application for federal funds to evaluation of program effectiveness, for which she received a FEMA Award for Exceptional Achievement.

FRED HENRETIG, M.D., is the Director of the Section of Clinical Toxicology at the Children's Hospital of Philadelphia, a Pediatric Specialist on a Disaster Medical Assistance Team of the National Disaster Medical System for the U.S. Public Health Service, and Professor of Pediatrics and Emergency Medicine at the University of Pennsylvania School of Medicine. He received his undergraduate education at University of Pennsylvania and an M.D. from Yale University School of Medicine. Dr. Henretig completed a residency in pediatrics at St. Christopher's Hospital for Children in Philadelphia. In his 25 years of pediatric emergency medicine, Dr. Henretig has achieved such honors as being elected twice to the American College of Medical Toxicology Board of Directors and being appointed to the American Board of Pediatrics' Medical Toxicology Subboard, which he chaired in 2000. Dr. Henretig's recent special interests include biological and chemical terrorism issues, and he has completed a six-month sabbatical at the U.S. Army's Medical Research Institute of Infectious Diseases with its biodefense group.

DARRELL HIGUCHI is Deputy Fire Chief, Service Bureau, County of Los Angeles Fire Department. He also serves as the department coordinator for the Terrorism Awareness and Preparedness Program, working closely with federal, state, and local government agencies including the Federal Bureau of Investigation, the Secret Service, and all branches of the armed forces. He is a member of the Interagency Board for Personal Protective Equipment and is the leader and administrator of the Los Angeles Metropolitan Medical Response System Task Force. Chief Higuchi began his 28 years on the County of Los Angeles Fire Department as a firefighter and paramedic and has held positions involving fire protection engineering, public affairs, and fire prevention. As Deputy Fire Chief for Operations, he was responsible for providing fire protection and emergency medical services to 31 cities and unincorporated areas of Los Angeles County. In his current position he commands the Fleet, Construction and Maintenance, and Command and Control Divisions, including the 911-command center and all communications equipment. Chief Higuchi is a graduate of California State University, Los Angeles, where he now holds an appointment as Associate Professor. He is a member of the International Association of Fire Chiefs, the National Fire Protection Association, and the American Association of Public Administration.

ARNOLD M. HOWITT, Ph.D., is Executive Director of the Taubman Center for State and Local Government at the John F. Kennedy School of Government, Harvard University. He also serves part-time as Executive Director of the Cooperative Mobility Program, an international transportation research program based at the Massachusetts Institute of Technology. Dr. Howitt specializes in state and local public management and intergovernmental relations. Currently, he is directing a multiyear study of transportation and air quality policy making in the federal government and in 15 states, supported in part by the U.S. Environmental Protection Agency and the Federal Highway Administration. He is also exploring transportation and air quality issues on an international basis, particularly in Japan and Mexico. In addition, Dr. Howitt is codirector of a new Kennedy School research project for the U.S. Department of Justice on domestic preparedness for terrorism. Dr. Howitt has authored books and chapters on the federal grant-in-aid system, management capacity building, the political economy of land use exactions, going private, transportation economics and policy, and state growth management regulatory programs. Several years ago, he coauthored *Stimulating Community Development*, a 3-year study of housing and economic development activities by neighborhood development organizations in Boston, Chicago, Cleveland, Indianapolis, Philadelphia, San Francisco, and the South Bronx. He also directed a national assessment of state government programs to promote labor-management cooperation in private industry. Dr. Howitt earned a B.A. from Columbia University and an M.A. and Ph.D. in political science from Harvard University. He has continuously served in faculty and administrative positions at Harvard since 1976, receiving the Fussa Distinguished Teaching Award from the Harvard Extension School in 1993. Since 1988, Dr. Howitt has also been a part-time faculty member at the Cascade Center for Public Service, Daniel J. Evans School of Public Affairs, University of Washington, Seattle. Previously, he was a faculty member at Brown University (1974–1976) and held a part-time appointment at the State University of New York at Albany (1984–1992). Dr. Howitt has extensive experience in executive education and has consulted with public agencies in several states and in the federal government.

LAURA LEVITON, Ph.D., is the Senior Program Officer for Research and Evaluation at the Robert Wood Johnson Foundation. Dr. Leviton received a B.A. degree in psychology at Reed College and an M.A. and Ph.D. in psychology from the University of Kansas and was a postdoctoral fellow in Research and Training in Evaluation of Social Programs at Northwestern University. Dr. Leviton has been appointed to CDC National Advisory Committee on HIV and STD Prevention of the Centers for Disease Control and Prevention and has served as chair for the National Review Committee of HIV Prevention Evaluation Grants for the state of California. She has published two books, 10 chapters, and 50 refereed publications. Dr. Leviton has won several awards including the Award for Distinguished Contributions to Psychology in the Public Interest from the

American Psychological Association. Dr. Leviton was a coinvestigator on the earliest and to date the largest randomized experiment on effective ways to prevent human immunodeficiency virus (HIV) infection in gay and bisexual men. She is coauthor of two books: *Foundations of Program Evaluation*, a dominant advanced evaluation research text, and *Confronting Public Health Risks*.

WILLIAM MYERS, M.S., retired from the post of Health Commissioner for the City of Columbus, Ohio, in February 2002 after 22 years of service in that role and 35 years of experience and knowledge in public health practice, planning principles, organizational change, communication, and developing community partnerships. Mr. Myers has an M.S. in preventive medicine from The Ohio State University and is a graduate of the Public Health Leadership Institute. He has held leadership positions with the National Association of County and City Health Officials and is a past president of the Ohio Public Health Association. Mr. Myers has served on national public health planning efforts and has made numerous presentations before nationwide bodies such as the National Commission on AIDS, the U.S. Conference of Mayors, and the American Public Health Association. Mr. Myers chaired the Columbus Metropolitan Medical Response System development committee. Mr. Myers believes in the principle that "all health is local" and has been an advocate for establishing local partnerships to help make Columbus the healthiest city in America.

DENNIS M. PERROTTA, Ph.D., C.I.C., is State Epidemiologist and Chief of the Bureau of Epidemiology, Texas Department of Health. He has a doctorate in epidemiology, is board certified in infection control, and has worked in public health for more than 20 years spanning a wide range of subject areas from bioterrorism, asthma, and environmental health to infectious disease epidemiology. Dr. Perrotta recently served as president of the Council of State and Territorial Epidemiologists and as president of the Armed Forces Epidemiological Board. From 1997 to 1999 he served on the Institute of Medicine's Committee to Improve Civilian Medical Response to Chemical and Biological Terrorism and is facilitating state health department efforts regarding bioterrorism preparedness. He is the principal investigator on a Centers for Disease Control and Prevention bioterrorism grant.

JEFFREY L. RUBIN is the Chief of the Disaster Medical Services Division for the Emergency Medical Services Authority for the state of California. He obtained a B.S. in business administration-finance at California State University and performed graduate work in health care administration. Mr. Rubin is responsible for the development and maintenance of plans, policies, and procedures governing state and local preparedness and response for major disasters involving mass casualties. He previously served as the manager of the EMT-Paramedic Licensure Program for the state of California and as a disaster medical program specialist and associate government program analyst.

AMY E. SMITHSON, Ph.D. (November 2000 to July 2001) is a Senior Associate at the Henry L. Stimson Center and since 1993 has directed the Chemical and Biological Weapons Nonproliferation Project, which serves as an information clearinghouse, watchdog, and problem solver regarding chemical and biological weapons issues. Under its auspices, Dr. Smithson has conducted analytical research across the spectrum of complex topics associated with the control and elimination of chemical and biological weapons. Her most recent research inventories the various federal response assets and training and equipment programs addressing domestic terrorism, airs widespread feedback from the front lines on these federal efforts, and shares innovative ideas from local emergency personnel on coordination, plans, tactics, and capabilities for dealing with these type of incidents. She has published widely in journals, testified before the U.S. Congress, and is frequently consulted by the national news media. Previously at the Stimson Center, she worked on proposals for the use of cooperative aerial inspections that would enhance arms control verification, confidence-building regimes, and peacekeeping efforts. At that time, she coedited *Open Skies, Arms Control, and Cooperative Security*. Dr. Smithson was also the principal investigator for a project that examined the suitability of the U.S. government's structure for addressing arms control issues in the post-Cold War era. Before joining the Stimson Center in 1990, she worked at Pacific-Sierra Research Corporation and the Center for Naval Analyses. She holds two bachelor's degrees, in political science and Russian, from the University of North Carolina, Chapel Hill, a master's in international relations from Georgetown University (1984), and a doctorate in political science from George Washington University.

DARREL STEPHENS is Chief of the Charlotte-Mecklenburg Police Department, Charlotte-Mecklenburg County, North Carolina. Chief Stephens was appointed Chief in September 1999. He was previously the City Administrator for the city of St. Petersburg, Florida. He also served as police chief in St. Petersburg from December 1992 to June 1997. He spent most of his career in policing, including over 6 years as the Executive Director of the Police Executive Research Forum, a Washington, D.C.-based association. He began his career in 1968 as a police officer with the Kansas City, Missouri, Police Department that included a 10-month visiting fellowship at the National Institute of Justice in 1972. He became the Assistant Police Chief in Lawrence, Kansas, in 1976 and in 1979 accepted the Largo, Florida, Police Chief position. In 1983 he became Chief of Police in Newport News, Virginia. He holds a B.S. in the administration of justice from the University of Missouri–Kansas City and an M.S. in public administration from Central Missouri State University.

IOM STAFF

FREDERICK J. MANNING, Ph.D., is a Senior Program Officer in Institute of Medicine's (IOM's) Board on Health Sciences Policy and study director. In 8 years at IOM, he has served as study director for projects addressing a variety of topics including medical isotopes, potential hepatitis drugs, blood safety and availability, rheumatic disease, resource sharing in biomedical research, occupational safety and health, and chemical and biological terrorism. Before joining IOM, Dr. Manning spent 25 years in the U.S. Army Medical Research and Development Command, serving in positions that included Director of Neuropsychiatry at the Walter Reed Army Institute of Research and Chief Research Psychologist for the Army Medical Department. Dr. Manning earned a Ph.D. in psychology from Harvard University in 1970, following undergraduate education at the College of the Holy Cross.

REBECCA LOEFFLER is a project assistant for the Evaluation of Metropolitan Medical Response Systems study. She earned a B.S. in psychology, with a minor in biology and a concentration in animal behavior, from James Madison University, Harrisonburg, Virginia.

ANDREW POPE, Ph.D., is director of the Board on Health Sciences Policy at the Institute of Medicine. With expertise in physiology and biochemistry, his primary interests focus on environmental and occupational influences on human health. Dr. Pope's previous research activities focused on the neuroendocrine and reproductive effects of various environmental substances on food-producing animals. During his tenure at the National Academy of Sciences and since 1989 at the Institute of Medicine, Dr. Pope has directed numerous studies on topics that include injury control, disability prevention, biologic markers, neurotoxicology, indoor allergens, and the enhancement of environmental and occupational health content in medical and nursing school curricula. Most recently, Dr. Pope directed studies on priority-setting processes at the National Institutes of Health, fluid resuscitation practices in combat casualties, and organ procurement and transplantation.

ALDEN CHANG is the administrative assistant for the Board on Health Sciences Policy. He began his career at the Institute of Medicine in February 1999 as project assistant for *Safe Work in the 21st Century* and has also worked on the *Organ Procurement and Transplantation: Assessing Current Policies and the Potential Impact of the DHHS Final Rule* study and the Forum on Emerging Infections. Mr. Chang earned a bachelor of arts degree in international relations from The George Washington University, Washington, D.C.

B
Selected Information About Federal Chemical, Biological, Radiological, Nuclear Consequence Management Response Teams (Appendix II, General Accounting Office Report GAO-01-14)

Response Team	Mission
Department of Defense	
Joint Task Force for Civil Support	Supports lead federal agency, establishes command and control of designated Department of Defense (DOD) forces, and provides military assistance to civil authorities to save lives, prevent human suffering, and provide temporary critical life support.
Chemical/Biological Rapid Response Team	Coordinates and integrates DOD's technical assistance for the neutralization, containment, dismantlement, and disposal of chemical or biological materials, and assists first responders in dealing with consequence management.
U.S. Army Technical Escort Unit	Provides chemical/biological advice, assessment, sampling, detection, field verification, packaging, escort, and render safe for chemical/biological devices or hazards.
U.S. Army Special Medical Augmentation Response Team—Nuclear/Biological/Chemical	Provides technical advice in the detection, neutralization, and containment of chemical, biological, or radiological hazardous materials in a terrorist event.
U.S. Army Special Medical Augmentation Response Team—Aero-Medical Isolation	Provides a rapid response evacuation unit to any area of the world to transport and provide patient care under conditions of biological containment to service members or U. S. civilians exposed to certain contagious and highly dangerous diseases.
U.S. Marine Corps Chemical-Biological Incident Response Force	Provides force protection or mitigation in the event of a terrorist incident, domestically or overseas.
U.S. Army Radiological Advisory Medical Team	Assists and furnishes radiological health hazard guidance to the on-scene commander or other responsible officials at an incident site and the installation medical authority.

Cited Authority	Number of Team (dedicated/collateral) Members and Team's Primary Location	Transportation Mode
Established Oct. 1, 1999 by Secretary of Defense directive.	Sixty dedicated personnel located at Fort Monroe, Va.	Travels by military aircraft or ground transportation. Initial team deploys within 4 hours.
Secretary of Defense directive based on the Defense Against Weapons of Mass Destruction Act of 1996 and Fiscal Year 1997 National Defense Authorization Act.	Fourteen dedicated personnel located at Aberdeen Proving Grounds, Md.	Travels by commercial or military aircraft or ground transportation. Initial team deploys within 4 hours, and remainder of team deploys in 10 to 12 hours.
Chemical Warfare Service directive dated Jan. 20, 1943.	One hundred ninety-three dedicated personnel located at Aberdeen Proving Grounds, Md.; Fort Belvoir, Va; Pine Bluff, Ark.; and Dugway, Ut.	Travels by military aircraft or ground transportation. Team deploys in 4 hours.
Established in 1998 by U.S. Army Surgeon General directive.	Six teams located at various sites with six collateral duty members per team.	Travels by military aircraft or ground transportation in 12 hours.
Established in 1977 by U.S. Army Surgeon General directive.	Approximately 20 collateral duty personnel at Fort Detrick, Md.	Travels by military aircraft.
Established in Apr. 1996 by the U.S. Marine Corps Commandant's planning guidance.	Three hundred seventy-three dedicated personnel at Indian Head, Md.	Travels by military aircraft or ground transportation. Initial team deploys in 6 hours, and remainder of team deploys in 24 hours.
Army Regulation 40-13, Feb. 1, 1985.	Eight to 10 collateral duty personnel located at Walter Reed Army Hospital, Washington, D.C.	Travels by military transportation, commercial aircraft, or personal vehicles within 8 hours.

Response Team	Mission
Department of Health and Human Services	
Management Support Teams	Manage federal medical teams and assets that are deployed in response to an incident.
National Medical Response Teams	Decontaminate casualties resulting from a hazardous materials incident, provide medical care, and deploy with pharmaceutical cache of antidotes and medical equipment.
Disaster Medical Assistance Teams	Provide emergency medical care during a disaster or other event.
Disaster Mortuary Operational Response Teams	Provide identification and mortuary services to state and local health officials upon request in the event of major disasters and emergencies.
National Pharmaceutical Stockpile	Resupplies state and local public health agencies with pharmaceuticals and other medical treatments in the event of a terrorist incident.

Cited Authority	Number of Team (dedicated/collateral) Members and Team's Primary Location	Transportation Mode
National Security Decision Directive 47, 1982; Federal Response Plan; Presidential Decision Directives 39 and 62.	Six to eight dedicated personnel located at Rockville, Md., supplemented by 18 to 20 collateral duty Department of Veterans Affairs personnel.	Travels by commercial or military aircraft. Initial team (2 to 5 members) expected to be ready to deploy within 2 hours and arrive within 12 hours. Full team expected to arrive within 12 to 24 hours.
Federal Response Plan; Presidential Decision Directives 39 and 62.	Four teams located at Washington, D.C. (non-deployable); Winston-Salem, N.C.; Denver, Colo.; and Los Angeles, Calif., with 36 collateral duty members per team.	Travels by commercial or military aircraft or ground transportation. Expected to be ready to deploy within 3 hours and arrive within 12 hours.
National Security Decision Directive 47; Public Health Service memorandum of understanding with each team and team sponsor; Federal Response Plan; Presidential Decision Directives 39 and 62.	Forty-four teams at various locations nationwide with 34 collateral duty members per team.	Travels by commercial or military aircraft or ground transportation. Expected to be ready to deploy within 3 to 4 hours and arrive within 12 to 24 hours.
Federal Response Plan; Presidential Decision Directives 39 and 62; Public Health Service/ National Association for Search and Rescue memorandum of understanding.	Ten teams at various locations nationwide with 25 to 31 collateral duty members per team.	Travels by commercial aircraft or ground transportation. Expected to be ready to deploy within 4 hours and at the site within 6 to 12 hours.
P.L. 105-277: Omnibus Consolidated and Emergency Appropriations Act of 1999.	Four to six dedicated personnel located at Atlanta, Ga.	Travels by commercial, charter, or military aircraft. Expected to arrive within 12 hours.

Response Team	Mission
Department of Energy	
Radiological Assistance Program Teams	Assist federal agencies, state and local governments, private business, or individuals in incidents involving radiological materials.
Federal Radiological Monitoring and Assessment Center[a]	Collects, evaluates, interprets, and distributes off-site radiological data in support of the lead federal agency, state and local governments. Coordinates federal resources in responding to the off-site monitoring and assessment needs at the scene of a radiological emergency.
Aerial Measuring System	Detects, measures, and tracks ground and airborne radioactivity over large areas using fixed-wing and rotary-wing aircraft.
Radiation Emergency Assistance Center/Training Site	Provides medical advice and on-site assistance in triage, diagnosis, and treatment of all types of radiation exposure events.
Department of Transportation	
U.S. Coast Guard National Strike Teams	Respond to oil and hazardous substance pollution incidents in and around waterways to protect public health and the environment. Area of responsibility includes all Coast Guard Districts and Federal Response Regions. Support Environmental Protection Agency's On-Scene Coordinators for inland area incidents.

Cited Authority	Number of Team (dedicated/collateral) Members and Team's Primary Location	Transportation Mode
Established in the late 1950s under the Atomic Energy Commission.	Twenty-six teams at various locations nationwide with seven collateral duty members per team.	Normally travels by ground transportation but can deploy by commercial aircraft. Expected to arrive within 2 to 6 hours.
Federal Radiological Emergency Response Plan.	Team members deploy in phases. Phases I (15 members) and II (45 members) consist of collateral duty Department of Energy personnel from Nellis Air Force Base, Nev., and other locations. Phase III (known as Full Federal Radiological Monitoring and Assessment Center) involves multiple federal agencies and may have 150 or more personnel from various federal agencies.	Travels by military, commercial, or Department of Energy-owned aircraft. Expected to arrive within 4 to 8 hours (phase I), 11 hours (phase II), and 24 to 36 hours (phase III).
Established in the early 1950s as a U.S. Geological Survey program to support the Atomic Energy Commission.	Five to 10 dedicated and collateral duty personnel located at Nellis Air Force Base, Nev., and Andrews Air Force Base, Md.	Initial team travels in fixed-wing aircraft and is expected to arrive within 4 to 8 hours.
Established in 1976 under an agreement between the Energy Research and Development Administration and a local hospital.	Four to eight dedicated personnel located in Oak Ridge, Tenn.	Travels by commercial or charter aircraft. Expected to be ready to deploy within 4 hours.
Federal Water Pollution Control Act of 1972; National Oil and Hazardous Substances Pollution Contingency Plan (40 C.F. R. 300); Oil Pollution Act of 1990.	Three teams located in Fort Dix, N.J.; Mobile, Ala.; and Novato, Calif., with 35 to 39 dedicated members per team.	Travels by military aircraft or ground transportation. Expected to deploy within 1 to 6 hours and arrive within 12 hours.

Response Team	Mission
U.S. Coast Guard On-Scene Coordinators	Coordinate all containment, removal and disposal efforts during a hazardous release incident in coastal or major navigational waterways.
Department of Veterans Affairs	
Medical Emergency Radiological Response Team	Provides technical advice, radiological monitoring, decontamination expertise, and medical care as a supplement to an institutional health care provider.
Environmental Protection Agency	
On-Scene Coordinators	Direct response efforts and coordinate all other efforts at the scene of a hazardous materials discharge or release.
Environmental Response Team	Provides technical support for assessing, managing, and disposing of hazardous waste.
Radiological Emergency Response Team	Provides mobile laboratories for field analysis of samples and technical expertise in radiation monitoring, radiation health physics, and risk assessment.

Cited Authority	Number of Team (dedicated/collateral) Members and Team's Primary Location	Transportation Mode
National Oil and Hazardous Substances Pollution Contingency Plan (40 C.F.R. 300).	Approximately 50 dedicated personnel in pre-designated Coast Guard regional zones at various locations nationwide.	Travels by ground transportation. On-call 24 hours. Response time depends on location of incident site.
Executive Order 12657: Federal Emergency Management Agency Assistance In Emergency Preparedness Planning at Commercial Nuclear Power Plants; Federal Radiological Emergency Response Plan.	Twenty-one to 23 collateral duty personnel are located at various sites nationwide.	Travels by commercial aircraft. Expected to be ready to deploy within 6 hours and arrive within 12 to 24 hours.
National Oil and Hazardous Substances Pollution Contingency Plan (40 C.F.R. 300).	Approximately 200 dedicated personnel, plus contractor support, at various locations nationwide.	Travels by commercial aircraft or ground transportation. Coordinators and contractors are on-call 24 hours. Response time depends on location of incident site.
National Oil and Hazardous Substances Pollution Contingency Plan (40 C.F.R. 300).	Twenty-two dedicated personnel, plus contractor support, located in Edison, N.J., and Cincinnati, Ohio.	Travels by commercial aircraft. Advance team expected to deploy within 4 hours. Full team expected to arrive within 24 to 48 hours.
National Oil and Hazardous Substances Pollution Contingency Plan (40 C.F.R. 300)	As many as 60 collateral duty personnel located in Las Vegas, Nev., and Montgomery, Ala.	Travels by ground transportation or military air. Expected to arrive within 2 to 3 days.

Response Team	Mission
Federal Emergency Management Agency	
Emergency Response Team	Coordinates federal response and recovery activities within a state.
Nuclear Regulatory Commission	
Regional Incident Response Teams	Carry out the responsibilities and functions of the lead federal agency during incidents at licensed facilities such as nuclear power plants.

[a] The Department of Energy has the lead responsibility for coordinating the Federal Radiological Monitoring Assessment Center during the early phase of an emergency. The Environmental Protection Agency assumes control during later phases.

Note: Agency officials define deployment time as the number of hours in which team members receive notification to leave for an incident and their arrival at their place of departure.

Cited Authority	Number of Team (dedicated/collateral) Members and Team's Primary Location	Transportation Mode
Robert T. Stafford Disaster Relief and Emergency Assistance Act, 42 U.S.C. 5121 et. seq.	Size is dependent on the severity and magnitude of the incident. Collateral duty team members are geographically dispersed at Federal Emergency Management Agency headquarters and 10 regional offices.	Travels by commercial, charter, or military aircraft, or ground transportation. Expected to arrive within 24 hours.
Public Law 96-295, dated June 30, 1980; Federal Radiological Emergency Response Plan.	Four teams located in Atlanta, Ga.; Lisle, Ill.; Arlington, Tex.; and King of Prussia, Penn., with 25 to 30 collateral duty members per team.	Travels by commercial or charter aircraft or ground transportation. Initial team expected to arrive within 6 to 12 hours.

They define arrival time as the number of hours in which the team is expected to reach the incident site after receiving notification. Department of Defense officials provided only deployment times for their teams.

Source: Our analysis and discussions with agency officials.

C

Metropolitan Medical Response System Program Cities

FISCAL YEAR 1996

Washington, DC, Atlanta

FISCAL YEAR 1997

Boston, New York, Baltimore, Philadelphia, Miami, Memphis, Jacksonville, Detroit, Chicago, Milwaukee, Indianapolis, Columbus (OH), San Antonio, Houston, Dallas, Kansas City (MO), Denver, Phoenix, San Jose, Honolulu, Los Angeles, San Diego, San Francisco, Anchorage, Seattle

FISCAL YEAR 1998

None

FISCAL YEAR 1999

El Paso, Cleveland, New Orleans, Nashville, Austin, Fort Worth, Oklahoma City, Portland, Long Beach, Tucson, St. Louis, Charlotte, Hampton Roads Area (Virginia Beach), Albuquerque, Oakland, Pittsburgh, Sacramento, Minneapolis, Tulsa, Salt Lake City

FISCAL YEAR 2000

Buffalo, Newark, Rochester, Jersey City, Hampton Roads Area (Norfolk),

Tampa, Louisville, Birmingham, St. Petersburg, Lexington-Fayette, Cincinnati, St. Paul, Toledo, Akron, Arlington (TX), Corpus Christi, Omaha, Wichita, Aurora, Fresno, Santa Ana, Mesa (AZ), Anaheim, Las Vegas, Riverside

FISCAL YEAR 2001

Colorado Springs, Baton Rouge, Raleigh, Stockton, Richmond (VA), Shreveport, Jackson, Mobile, Des Moines, Lincoln, Madison, Grand Rapids, Yonkers, Hialeah, Montgomery, Lubbock, Greensboro, Dayton, Huntington Beach, Garland, Glendale (CA), Columbus (GA), Spokane, Tacoma, Little Rock

FISCAL YEAR 2002

Bakersfield, Fremont, Ft. Wayne, Hampton Roads Area (Newport News), Arlington (VA), Worcester, Knoxville, Modesto, Orlando, San Bernardino, Syracuse, Providence, Huntsville, Amarillo, Springfield (MA), Irving (TX), Chattanooga, Hampton Roads Area (Chesapeake), Kansas City (KS), Jefferson Parish (LA), Ft. Lauderdale, Glendale (AZ), Warren (MI), Hartford (CT), Columbia (SC)

D

2000 MMRS Contract Deliverable Evaluation Instrument

2000 MMRS Contract Deliverable Evaluation Instrument

City Evaluated: ________________________

Evaluator: ________________________

Date Complete: ________________________

01 Deliverable #1: Meeting with Project Officer.

Contract Reference: (2000 Statement of Work #1)

Meet with Project Officer to discuss the purpose of this contract and review key aspects of the accepted proposal. This meeting to be held not more than one month after the award of the contract. (2000 Statement of Work #1)

Indicators of Fulfillment:

01.01 Did the contracted city meet with the project officer to discuss the purpose of the contract and review key aspects of the accepted proposal within 1 month of the award of the contract?

01.02 Notes:

02 Deliverable #2: MMRS Development Plan.

Contract Reference: (2000 Statement of Work #2)

Create a MMRS Development Plan to outline the approach to the creation of an enhanced ability to deal with a terrorist use of a weapon of mass destruction (WMD), and to identify how the Public Safety, Public Health, and Health Services sector responses to an N/B/C terrorist incident will be coordinated. This MMRS Development Plan should detail the proposed leadership and membership of the development team and the philosophy underlying the proposed approach, along with a description of the geographic area that the plan will cover. The plan must also include a roster of the Steering Committee membership, representing the relevant organizations, that will assist in the planning and development of the MMRS. Consideration should be given to the following Steering Committee membership: EMS, EMS Project Medical Directors, public and private hospital representation, hospital ER representation from major receiving hospitals, Local and State Emergency Management, Local Emergency Planning Committees (LEPCs), National Guard, Local and State Public Health departments (infectious disease representation), Mental Health, 911, Poison Control Centers, Medical Examiner, local lab representation, Police/FBI (including bomb squad), American Red Cross, and local federal agency representatives (i.e., DoD, VA, DOE, EPA, FEMA) where available. This development plan shall be completed in consultation with the Project Officer not more than three months after contract award. (2000 Statement of Work #2)

Indicators of Fulfillment:

02.01 Does the plan indicate that the MMRS represents an enhanced ability to deal with a terrorist use of a WMD?

02.02 Does the plan identify how the Public Safety, Public Health, and Health Services sector responses to an N/B/C terrorist incident will be coordinated?

02.03 Does the plan detail the proposed leadership and membership of the development team?

02.04 Does the plan detail the philosophy underlying the proposed approach?

02.05 Does the plan contain a description of the geographic area that the plan will cover?

02.06 Does the plan include a roster of the Steering Committee membership, representing the relevant organizations, which will assist in the planning and development of the MMRS? (i.e., Command & Control, MMST or Capability, Emergency Patient Transportation, Hospital Emergency Services, Mental Health Services, Mass Fatality Management, Forward Movement via NDMS.)

02.07 Is the Steering Committee membership inclusive of a broad base of emergency response disciplines? (i.e., EMS, EMS Project Medical Directors, public and private hospital representation, hospital ER representation from major receiving hospitals, Local and State Emergency Management, Local Emergency Planning Committees [LEPCs], National Guard, Local and State Public Health departments infectious disease representation, Mental Health, 911, Poison Control Centers, Medical Examiner, local lab representation, Police/FBI [including bomb squad], American Red Cross, and local federal agency representatives [i.e., DoD, VA, DOE, EPA, FEMA] where available)

02.08 Has the MMRS development plan been completed in consultation with the Project Officer not more than three months of contract award?

02.09 Notes:

03 Deliverable #3: Primary MMRS Plan.

Contract Reference: (2000 Statement of Work #3)

Develop a Primary Metropolitan Medical Response System (MMRS) Plan for managing the human health consequences of a terrorist incident involving the use of weapons of mass destruction (WMD), i.e., a nuclear, radiological, biological and/or chemical device capable of creating mass casualties. *The MMRS is considered to be an enhanced local capability for an existing system.* The MMRS plan must interface with the State plan, and should be coordinated with other appropriate political jurisdictions (e.g., county government), with nearby/neighboring emergency response systems, and with nearby/neighboring MMRS systems (within approximately 25 miles or those with whom mutual aid is anticipated to be used). This plan should identify and accommodate resident Federal/State assets that may be useful for the city/metropolitan area response plan. The MMRS should develop plans: for command and control, for notification and alert procedures, for management of public affairs, for provision of accurate and timely information, for centralized communication control, for control of transportation assets, for management/augmentation of medical personnel, for management of medical supplies and equipment, for emergency management of legal issues and credentialing, for emergency management of patient tracking/record keeping, for augmentation of epidemiological services and support, for laboratory support, for crowd control, protection of treatment facilities and personnel, for establishing a schedule for exercises, and for assigning responsibility for afteraction reports and addressing report findings. Mental health services should be designed for the care of emergency workers, victims and their families as well as others in the community who need special assistance in coping with the consequences of this type of event. Plans for the proper examination, care and disposition of any humans that do not survive the attack should be included. A completed plan, including the preceding, must be submitted to the Project Officer not more than six months after contract award. (2000 Statement of Work #3)

Indicators of Fulfillment:

03.01 Does the plan detail the development of an MMRS for managing the human health consequences of a terrorist incident involving the use of a WMD?

03.02 Does the plan identify that the MMRS is considered an enhanced local capability for an existing system?

03.03 Does the plan interface with the State plan?

03.04 Has the plan been coordinated with other appropriate political, mutual aid, or other MMRS development jurisdictions (within approximately 25 miles)?

03.05 Does the plan identify and accommodate resident Federal/ State assets that may be useful for the city/metropolitan area response plan?

03.06 Does the plan identify command and control measures?

03.07 Does the plan detail notification and alert procedures?

03.08 Does the plan detail the management of public affairs?

03.09 Does the plan include provisions for accurate and timely information?

03.10 Does the plan establish centralized communications control?

03.11 Does the plan establish the control of transportation assets?

03.12 Does the plan detail the management/augmentation of medical personnel?

03.13 Does the plan detail the management of medical supplies and equipment?

03.14 Does the plan provide for emergency management of legal issues and credentialing?

03.15 Does the plan provide for emergency management of patient tracking/record keeping?

03.16 Does the plan provide for augmentation of epidemiological services and support?

03.17 Does the plan provide for laboratory support?

03.18 Does the plan provide for crowd control?

03.19 Does the plan provide for protection of treatment facilities and personnel?

03.20 Does the plan establish a schedule for exercises?

03.21 Does the plan assign responsibility for after-action reports and addressing report findings?

03.22 Does the plan designate mental health services to care for emergency workers, victims and their families, and others in the community who need special assistance in coping with the consequences of a WMD event?

03.23 Does the plan provide for the proper examination, care and disposition of any humans that do not survive the attack?

03.24 Has a Primary MMRS plan been submitted to the Project Officer not more than 6 months of contract award?

03.25 Notes:

04 Deliverable #4: Component MMRS Plan for forward movement of patients utilizing the NDMS System.

Contract Reference: (2000 Statement of Work #4)

To the extent that local resources are insufficient to provide the definitive health care required for all of those directly affected by the attack, develop a component of the MMRS Plan for Forward Movement of Patients to other areas of the region or nation. An important consideration here is; who will make the decision to implement the forward movement of patients? This transportation and care would be provided by the National Disaster Medical System (this plan should be developed in coordination with the applicable Federal Coordinating Hospital FCH). These plans outlining how the contractor is going to accomplish the preceding shall be completed in consultation with the Project Officer within eight months of the award of the contract. (2000 Statement of Work #4)

Indicators of Fulfillment:

04.01 Does the Component MMRS Plan detail how patients are prepared for forward movement to other areas of the region or nation?

04.02 Does the Component MMRS Plan identify who will make the decision to implement the forward movement of patients?

04.03 Does the Component MMRS Plan indicate that the National Disaster Medical System would provide transportation and care?

04.04 Has the Component MMRS Plan for forward movement of patients utilizing the National Disaster Medical System been completed in consultation with the Project Officer within eight months of contract award?

04.05 Notes:

05 Deliverable #5: Component MMRS Plan for responding to a chemical, radiological, nuclear, or explosive WMD event.

Contract Reference: (2000 Statement of Work #5)

Develop a component of the MMRS Plan for responding to and managing the health consequences of an incident resulting from the use of a chemical, radiological, nuclear, and explosive WMD. The MMRS should be able to detect and identify the weapon material or agent, extract the victims, administer the appropriate antidote, decontaminate victims, triage them and provide primary care prior to their transportation to a definitive medical care facility. The MMRS shall include plans for emergency medical transportation of the patients as well as emergency and inpatient services in hospitals that have the capacity and capability to provide the definitive medical care required, or to pre-designated off-site treatment facilities. Management of patients arriving at hospitals without prior field treatment/screening or decontamination should also be part of the MMRS. This plan shall also include procurement and provision of appropriate pharmaceuticals (sufficient to provide care for up to 1,000 victims), equipment, and supplies consistent with the mission and the MMRS. A completed plan, including the preceding, must be submitted to the Project Officer not more than 9 months after contract award. No pharmaceuticals or antidotes may be purchased until the list has been submitted to, and approved by, the Project Officer. (2000 Statement of Work #5)

Indicators of Fulfillment:

05.01 Does the Component MMRS Plan identify procedures for the effective management of the health consequences of an incident resulting from the use of a chemical, radiological, nuclear, or explosive WMD?

05.02 Does the Component MMRS Plan include detailed procedures for detecting and identifying the weapon material or agent?

05.03 Does the Component MMRS Plan include detailed procedures for extracting victims?

05.04 Does the Component MMRS Plan include detailed procedures for administering appropriate antidotes?

05.05 Does the Component MMRS Plan include detailed procedures for decontamination of victims?

05.06 Does the Component MMRS Plan identify the procedures for victim triage and procedures for providing primary care prior to transportation to a definitive medical care facility?

05.07 Does the Component MMRS Plan include provisions for the emergency medical transportation of victims?

05.08 Does the Component MMRS Plan provide for emergency and impatient services in hospitals that have the capacity and capability to provide the definitive medical care required, or in pre-designated off-site treatment facilities?

05.09 Does the Component MMRS Plan include procedures for managing patients arriving at hospitals without prior field treatment/screening or decontamination?

05.10 Does the Component MMRS Plan provide for procurement and provision of appropriate pharmaceuticals sufficient to provide care for up to 1,000 victims?

05.11 Does the Component MMRS Plan identify procurement and provision of appropriate equipment and supplies consistent with the mission and the MMRS?

05.12 Has the Component MMRS Plan for responding to a chemical, radiological, nuclear, or explosive WMD event been submitted to the Project Officer within 9 months of contract award?

06. Deliverable #6: Component Plan for MMST if it is a component of your MMRS. (Optional)

Contract Reference: (2000 Statement of Work #6)

If a clearly identifiable Metropolitan Medical Strike Team (MMST) is a component of your MMRS plan, develop a component of the MMRS Plan for MMST capability that includes its mission statement, organization, membership, and concept of operations. Included in this operational plan shall be provisions for its activation, deployment, N/B/C agent identification, extraction of victims from the incident site, antidote administration, human decontamination, triage and primary care, and preparation of victims for transportation to definitive care facilities with sufficient supplies of appropriate antidotes to assure adequate treatment. This plan shall be submitted to the Project Officer no later than 12 months after the award of the contract. (2000 Statement of Work #6)

Indicators of Fulfillment:

06.01 Does the Component MMRS Plan contain a mission statement and concept of operations for the MMST?

06.02 Does the Component MMRS Plan detail the organization and membership of the MMST?

06.03 Does the Component MMRS Plan detail procedures for the activation and deployment of the MMST?

06.04 Does the Component MMRS Plan detail procedures for the identification of the agent?

06.05 Does the Component MMRS Plan detail procedures for extraction of victims from the incident site?

06.06 Does the Component MMRS Plan detail procedures for administration of appropriate antidote?

06.07 Does the Component MMRS Plan detail procedures for human decontamination?

06.08 Does the Component MMRS Plan detail provisions for triage and primary care of victims?

06.09 Does the Component MMRS Plan detail preparation of victims for transportation to definitive care facilities with sufficient supplies of appropriate antidotes to assure adequate treatment?

06.10 Has the Component MMRS Plan been submitted to the Project Officer within 12 months of contract award?

06.11 Notes:

07 Deliverable #7: Component Plan for managing the health consequences of a biological WMD.

Contract References: (2000 Statement of Work #7 and Contract APPENDIX B)

Develop a component of the MMRS Plan to manage the health consequences of the release of a biological weapon of mass destruction. This plan should be integrated with existing or planned Local and State health surveillance plans for bioterrorism and influenza pandemic planning. This portion of the plan should address five general areas. (1) Early Recognition: the contractor should identify, describe, or develop "early warning indicator(s)" which will be used to alert local officials of a biological terrorist event, ensuring timely notification and activation of response plans. This plan should identify who will receive notification, and who will make the decision to further implement response plans. (2) Mass Immunization/Prophylaxis: In this section, the contractor should highlight, develop, or augment existing plans for managing and implementing mass immunization I prophylaxis. In developing this plan, it should be assumed that the Federal government would assure the availability of vaccines and antibiotics within 24 hours of notification. Key components of this plan include a description of the decision making process to initiate a mass immunization campaign, together with plans for identifying the affected population. (3) Mass Patient Care: In this section, the contractor should develop or augment existing plans for providing care for a significant portion of the population. Key components of this plan include plans for rapid expansion of existing healthcare system capacity, and plans for taking care of people in excess of either existing or expanded capacity. (4) Mass Fatality Management: In this section, the contractor should develop or augment existing plans for providing respectful care and disposition for a large percentage of the population. Key components of this plan are plans for augmenting existing morgue facilities and staff, and plans for decontamination/isolation procedures where appropriate. (5) Environmental Surety: In this section, the contractor should describe or develop a plan for identifying environmental risk, need for decontamination or vector intervention, and a process for safe re-entry into a suspect area in consultation with local, state, and federal environmental agencies. This concept of operations and related plans must be submitted to the Project Officer no later than 18 months after the award of the contract. (2000 Statement of Work #7)

The size and robustness of any response to the use of a biological weapon of mass destruction (WMD) will be determined by the specific biological agent. As a result, response planning should be considered at three (3) levels: 1. incidents with up to one hundred (100) victims, 2. incidents with one hundred (100) to ten thousand (10,000) victims, 3. incidents with more than ten thousand (10,000) victims. (2000 Statement of Work #7)

A list of Biological Agents that should be considered is: Smallpox, Anthrax, Plague, Botulism, Tularemia, and Hemorrhagic Fever. (2000-Contract-APPENDIX B)

Indicators of Fulfillment:

07.01 Is the Component MMRS Plan integrated with existing Local and State health surveillance plans for bioterrorism and influenza pandemic planning?

07.02 Does the Component MMRS Plan identify the five general areas: Early Recognition, Mass Immunization/Prophylaxis, Mass Patient Care, Mass Fatality Management, and Environmental Surety?

07.03 Does the Component MMRS Plan identify, describe, or develop early warning indicators that will be used to alert local officials of a biological terrorist event?

07.04 Does the Component MMRS Plan identify who will receive notification and who will make the decision to further implement response plans?

07.05 Does the Component MMRS Plan highlight, develop, or augment existing plans for management and implementation of mass immunization/prophylaxis?

07.06 Does the Component MMRS Plan include a description of the decision making process to initiate a mass immunization campaign and accomplish identification of the affected population?

07.07 Does the Component MMRS Plan develop or augment existing plans for providing care for a significant portion of the population?

07.08 Does the Component MRS Plan detail procedures for rapid expansion of the existing health care system capacity, and plans for taking care of people in excess of either existing or expanded capacity?

07.09 Does the Component MRS Plan develop or augment existing mass fatality management plans for providing respectful care and disposition for a large percentage of the population?

07.10 Does the Component MRS Plan detail procedures for augmenting existing morgue facilities and staff?

07.11 Does the Component MRS Plan detail procedures for decontamination/isolation of human remains where appropriate?

07.12 Does the Component MRS Plan describe or develop procedures for identifying environmental risk, and determining the need for decontamination or vector intervention?

07.13 Does the Component MRS Plan establish a process for safe reentry into the affected area in consultation with Local, State, and Federal environmental agencies?

07.14 Does the Component MRS Plan provide for three levels of response: up to 100 victims, between 100 and 10,000 victims, and more than 10,000 victims?

07.15 Has the Component MRS Plan for managing the health consequences of a biological WMD been submitted to the Project Officer within 18 months of contract award?

07.16 Notes:

08 Deliverable #8: Component Plan for local hospital and healthcare system plan.

Contract Reference: (2000 Statement of Work #8)

Develop a component of the MMRS Plan for the local hospital and healthcare system. Current JCAHO standards for emergency preparedness address an emergency preparedness management plan (EC.1.6), a security management plan (EC.1.4), a hazardous materials and waste management plan (EC.1.5), and emergency preparedness drills (EC.2.9). Ensure that this portion of the plan addresses the following eight general areas. (1) Plans for notification of hospitals, clinics, HMOs, etc. that an incident has occurred. (2) Plans and procedures in place for hospitals, clinics, and HMOs to protect them from contamination from environmental or patient sources. (3) Plans for providing triage and initiation of definitive care at local healthcare facilities. (4) Plans for adequate security to support these activities. (5) Availability of adequate personal protective equipment for hospital and clinic providers. (6) Adequate pharmaceuticals and equipment (ventilators) are available locally, or that plans are in place to obtain them in a timely manner. (7) Ability of medical staff to recognize and treat casualties caused by WMD agents. (8) Treatment protocols are readily available. These plans shall be presented to the Project Officer no later than 18 months after award of the contract. (2000 Statement of Work #8)

Indicators of Fulfillment:

08.01 Does the Component MMRS plan detail procedures for notification of hospitals, clinics, HMOs, etc. that an incident has occurred?

08.02 Does the Component MMRS plan identify procedures in place to protect hospitals, clinics, and HMOs from contamination from environmental or patient sources (lock-down procedures)?

08.03 Does the Component MMRS plan detail that local healthcare facilities are capable of providing triage and initiation of definitive care?

08.04 Does the Component MMRS plan include the existence of adequate security to support these activities?

08.05 Does the Component MMRS plan identify the availability of adequate personal protective equipment for hospital and clinic providers?

08.06 Does the Component MMRS plan specify that adequate pharmaceuticals and equipment (ventilators) are available locally, or that plans are in place to obtain them in a timely manner?

08.07 Does the Component MMRS plan specify that medical staff can recognize and treat casualties caused by WMD agents?

08.08 Does the Component MMRS plan detail that treatment protocols are readily available?

08.09 Has the Component MMRS plan been submitted to the Project Officer within 18 months of contract award?

08.10 Notes:

09 Deliverable #9: MMRS Training Plan to include training requirements and a follow-on training plan.

Contract Reference: (2000 Statement of Work #9)

Develop a Training Plan for the MRS that identifies training requirements for MRS personnel, including all first responders EMTs, paramedics, vehicle drivers, emergency room and other hospital personnel who will be providing care to victims of a WMD incident. In the event that the DOD Domestic Preparedness training has been provided to the city, the contractor should indicate how the training received, including FEMA/DOJ training, will be integrated into meeting the initial training requirements as well as continuing education and other refresher training needs. For the training of hospital personnel, it is important to note that Presidential Decision Directive 62 (PDD 62) highlights the VA's role in the training of medical personnel in NDMS hospitals. This plan shall be presented to the Project Officer no later than 18 months after award of the contract. (2000 Statement of Work #9)

Indicators of Fulfillment:

09.01 Does the plan identify training requirements for MRS personnel, including all first responders EMTs, paramedics, vehicle drivers, emergency room and other hospital personnel who will be providing care to victims of a WMD incident?

09.02 Does the plan indicate how previously received training will be integrated into meeting initial training requirements as well as continuing education and other refresher training needs?

09.03 Does the plan highlight the VA's role in the training of medical personnel in NDMS hospitals?

09.04 Has the plan for identifying training requirements along with training plan been submitted to the Project Officer no later than 18 months of contract award?

09.05 Notes:

10 Deliverable #10: MRS Pharmaceutical and Equipment Plan that includes a maintenance plan and a procurement timetable for equipment and pharmaceuticals to be purchased after receipt of Project Officer approval.

Contract Reference: (2000 Statement of Work #10)

Develop MRS Pharmaceutical and Equipment Plans. Submit a list of pharmaceuticals consistent with the mission of the MMRS. Pharmaceuticals should be sufficient to provide care for at least 1,000 victims, for a chemical incident, and for the affected population for the first 24 hours of response for a biological incident. (It should be assumed that the Federal government would assure the availability of vaccines and antibiotics within 24 hours of notification.) Equipment may include personal protective equipment, detection equipment and decontamination equipment (both field and hospital). A timetable for procurement of the above items and a plan for equipment maintenance and pharmaceutical storage should accompany this. A property officer responsible for all property received and purchased under this contract shall be identified. Equipment purchases under this contract must be harmonized with equipment received from DoD, DOJ, and FEMA programs. Only equipment and pharmaceuticals approved by the Project Officer shall be purchased under this contract. These plans shall be presented to the Project Officer no later than 18 months after the award of the contract. (2000 Statement of Work #10)

Indicators of Fulfillment:

10.01 Is the list of pharmaceuticals consistent with the mission of the MMRS?

10.02 Are the pharmaceuticals sufficient to provide care for at least 1,000 victims, for a chemical incident, and for the affected population for the first 24 hours of response for a biological incident?

10.03 Does the plan contain a timetable for procurement of pharmaceuticals and equipment?

10.04 Does the plan detail procedures for equipment maintenance and pharmaceutical storage?

10.05 Does the plan identify a property officer who is responsible for all property received and purchased under this contract?

10.06 Are equipment purchases under this contract harmonized with equipment received from DoD, DOJ, and FEMA programs?

10.07 Has the plan been submitted to the Project Officer no later than 18 months of contract award?

10.08 Notes:

11 Deliverable #11: Progress Reports (brief monthly status reports) and Final Report.

Contract Reference: (2000 Statement of Work #11)

Provide monthly progress reports (three copies), to be received by the 15th of the month that describe activities undertaken the previous month. These reports should be sent to your project officer, the PSC Contracting Officer, and to the Office of Emergency Preparedness (names and address will be provided). These reports should describe successful endeavors and barriers encountered. Any barrier encountered should be accompanied with a plan to resolve the issue. Include all meeting minutes that relate to MMRS development. A final report is due at the end of the 18-month contract period. (2000 Statement of Work #11)

Indicators of Fulfillment:

11.01 Has the contracted city submitted monthly progress reports describing successful endeavors and barriers encountered?

11.02 If a barrier was identified in the report, was a plan included to resolve the issue?

11.03 Do the monthly reports include all meeting minutes that relate to MMRS development?

11.04 Has the contracted city submitted a final report at the end of the contract period?

11.05 Notes:

12 Deliverable #12 (Option Period): Continue Progress Reports. Detailed list of pharmaceutical and equipment acquisition. Final Operational Report (include addendum to Primary MMRS Plan).

Contract Reference: (2000 Statement of Work #12)

Carry out remaining actions that are required to assure that the MMRS is operational, including acquisition of pharmaceuticals and equipment as identified, planned and approved in deliverable #10. Continue to submit brief monthly progress reports and a final report at the end of this contract period. The final report must constitute an assessment of response capabilities (enhanced or created), that exist now as a result of the MMRS planning effort. The report must identify actual equipment and pharmaceuticals procured and received under this contract. Identify additional assets/requirements that you will look to the Federal government to provide. These additional assets must be addressed in an addendum to your Primary MMRS Plan. The final report must include a statement that the MMRS has demonstrated operational capability. This final report shall be presented to the Project Officer no later than 12 months from the effective date of the Option Period. (2000 Statement of Work #12)

Indicators of Fulfillment:

12.01 Does the final report include a statement that the MMRS has demonstrated operational capability?

12.02 Does the final report identify actual equipment and pharmaceuticals procured and received under this contract?

12.03 Does the final report contain or include an assessment of response capabilities (enhanced or created) that exist now as a result of the MMRS planning effort?

12.04 Does the Primary MMRS plan include an addendum identifying additional assets/requirements that the contracted city will look to the Federal government to provide?

12.05 Has the final report been submitted to the Project Officer no later than 12 months from the effective date of the Option Period?

12.06 Did the final report include an electronic copy in Microsoft Word format?

12.07 Notes:

E
Preparedness Indicators for Metropolitan Medical Response System Program Contract Deliverables

Deliverable 2: MMRS Development Plan

Plan Elements	Inputs
2.02 Description of how responses to a chemical, biological, or radiological (CBR) terrorism incident by public safety, public health, and health services sectors will be coordinated	–List of relevant safety and health organizations –Description of proposed mechanisms for coordination of responses –Designation of lead agency or official
2.03 Identification of leadership and membership of the developmental team	–List of relevant safety and health organizations
2.New 1 Description of the planning environment	–Plan for soliciting input or gathering data
2.04 Statement of the philosophy of approach	–Mission or vision statement
2.05 Description of the geographic area	–Map of metropolitan area or list of jurisdictions in metropolitan area
2.06 and 2.07 Inclusion on steering committee of all relevant organizations, including broad base of organizations from emergency response disciplines	–Representation by senior officials from public safety, public health, and health care communities –Organizational tables and contact numbers
2.New 2 Periodic review of membership, gaps in planning, execution of plan, and response to CBR agent-related terrorism and proxy incidents	–Schedule of reviews

Processes	Outputs
–Meeting minutes –Draft documents and letters –Agreement to participate attested to by signature of the deliverable by representatives from each participating organization	–Demonstration of effective coordination in an exercise or documentation of effective coordination in an actual incident with or without CBR agents
–Sign-off by appropriate officials –Designation of lead individual or official and contact information (point of contact [POC]) for each organization –Memorandum of understanding (MOU) or other formal written agreement where appropriate	–Ability of designated officials to talk knowledgeably about their agency's role in the MMRS plan
–Evidence of ongoing analysis of community strengths, weaknesses, opportunities, and threats	–Identified strengths, barriers, and challenges –Priority list for planning efforts –List of designated officials and agencies and deadlines for each effort
	–Ability of representatives from different levels of key institutions to explain mission or vision statement to peer reviewer
–Written commitment by participating jurisdictions and state officials –Designation of lead individual or official and contact information for each jurisdiction	–Map or list of participating jurisdictions –See entry for proposed new plan element, Description of the planning environment
–Evidence of attendance and participation in steering committee meetings by representatives from public safety, public health, and health care communities (e.g., minutes)	–Written or oral guidance to drafters of the MMRS plan components
–Meeting minutes	–Restructured coordinating committee as required –File of periodic and after-action evaluations –Reports on quality and system improvements

Deliverable 3: Primary MMRS Plan

Plan Elements	Inputs
3.02 Indication of existing system(s) being enhanced	–Relevant pre-MMRS disaster plans, emergency operations plans, hazmat procedures, and state and local laws and regulations
3.03 Establishment of interfaces with state plan	–State plan –State plan POC
3.04 Coordination with other political, mutual-aid, or other MMRS program jurisdictions	–List of other relevant agencies in local jurisdictions, with POCs
3.05 Identification and plan for accommodating resident federal assets of potential use	–List of resident or neighboring federal assets, with POCs
3.06 Identification of command-and-control measures	–Description of current command-and-control measures
3.07 Detailed notification and alert procedures	–MMRS communication plans (telephone and fax numbers, e-mail addresses, radio frequencies and call signs, etc.)
3.08 Detailed management procedures for public affairs	–Designated spokesperson(s) and media plan –List of topics for preplanned media packages –List of news media outlets, including those serving non-English speakers and those with impaired sight or hearing –Protocols for media credentialing

Processes	Outputs
–Identification of gaps and shortfalls of existing plans –Designation of officials or agencies to address identified gaps and shortfalls	–Goals and objectives for enhancing existing plans
–Meeting minutes, e-mail, and other evidence of interaction with state POC –Sign-off on MMRS plan by state plan POC	–Alterations in state plan or functioning reflecting MMRS planning –Evidence from exercises or actual events demonstrating workable interface between local and state plans
–Meeting minutes, e-mail, and other evidence of interaction with local POCs –Sign-off on MMRS plan by local POCs	–Alterations in plans or functioning of other local jurisdictions reflecting MMRS planning –Evidence from exercises or actual events demonstrating workable interface among local plans
–Meeting minutes, e-mail, and other evidence of interaction with POCs of local federal facilities during the planning process –Sign-off on MMRS program plan by POCs of local federal facilities, with MOUs, where appropriate	–Evidence of involvement of federal partners in tabletop or field exercises and other emergency response activities
–Enhancements or revisions to command-and-control measures for MMRS plan, if needed –Distribution of identified measures to affected agencies	–Evidence (documentation or as a result of an actual incident with or without CBR agents) of agreement that all affected agencies have agreed to integration into a command structure that in some instances will make them subordinate to a sister agency
–Periodic testing, including during all shifts and under adverse conditions (during holidays, storms, etc.)	–Documented success in regular testing or actual use in an emergency
–Draft or incomplete set of communiqués for news media on agents, procedures, and public safety –Arrangements for backup communication systems through state emergency management agency or law enforcement channels	–Collection of finished communiqués –Documented use of media packages in CBR agent-related hoaxes or incidents or other hazmat or epidemic events

Deliverable 3: Continued

Plan Elements	Inputs
3.09 Provisions for accurate and timely dissemination of information among MMRS members	–List of current and planned communication systems, including telephone and pager numbers, radio frequencies and call signs, and Internet or intranet addresses of all participating organizations –Standard operating procedures (SOPs) describing when and how to use basic equipment –Equipment and procedures for communication in conditions in which demand or infrastructure damage may make public systems unreliable or unavailable
3.10 Provisions for centralized communications control	–See 3.09
3.11 Provisions for control of transportation assets, medical and nonmedical	–List of available sources for vehicles and drivers, including those available through mutual-aid agreements, state agencies, and local federal institutions –SOPs for accessing assets
3.12 Detailed procedures for the management and augmentation of medical personnel	–Collection of staff augmentation plans –List of sources of additional medical personnel, with POCs
3.13 Provisions for management of medical supplies and equipment (see also Deliverable 10)	–Communitywide list of routine inventory by location –See Deliverable 10
3.14 Provisions for emergency management of legal issues and credentialing	–POCs for legal affairs –Clear explanation of legal status and liability of medical and other personnel, including volunteers, responding as part of the MMRS program –Copies of or reference to relevant laws and regulations –Procedure for requesting emergency waivers or exceptions

Processes	Outputs
–Evidence of dissemination to all relevant organizations –Record or schedule of system checks or tests	–Demonstration of effective use of all systems in periods of peak demand through unannounced tests or use in an actual emergency
–See 3.09	–See 3.09
–Evidence of periodic communication with managers of assets	–Demonstration of availability of anticipated assets on short notice for random check, planned exercise, or actual emergency
–Communitywide list of augmentation personnel, without duplicates –Record or schedule of system checks	–Demonstration of effective use of all systems at multiple sites, for several types of medical personnel, and in periods of peak demand through unannounced tests or use in an actual emergency (snowstorm, hurricane, etc.) –Documented resolution of any issues related to cross-jurisdictional licensure and liability coverage
–Periodic assessment of actual inventory –See Deliverable 10	–See Deliverable 10
–Confirmation of MMRS plan description of legal issues by legal POCs –Evidence that efforts are under way to eliminate legal obstacles to preparedness	–Confirmation by legal authorities that MMRS plans conform to local, state, and federal laws (e.g., the Emergency Medical Treatment and Labor Act)

Deliverable 3: Continued

Plan Elements	Inputs
3.15 Provisions for emergency management of patient tracking and record keeping	–MMRS plan
3.16 Provisions for augmentation of epidemiological services and support	–List of supporting agencies or institutions, with POCs
3.17 Provisions for laboratory support	–List of supporting agencies or institutions, with POCs
3.18 Provisions for crowd control	–MMRS plan –List of available law enforcement and security assets, with POCs
3.19 Provisions for protection of treatment facilities and personnel	–Same as 3.18
3.20 A schedule for exercises	–Inclusion on the schedule of an exercise of all required MMRS program functions, separately or together, at least on a yearly basis –Inclusion on the schedule of a full-scale field exercise at least every 2 years
3.21 Assignment of responsibility for after-action reports and addressing report findings	–Name(s) of designated individual(s)

Processes	Outputs
–Evidence of implementation of patient tracking plan, software, and training at health care facilities in metropolitan area (e.g., meeting minutes, purchases, training log)	–Demonstration of effective patient tracking in an exercise or a multiple-casualty incident of any sort involving large-scale movement of patients within and across health care facilities
–Evidence of interaction with and input to planning by POCs –Sign-off or other evidence of agreement with MMRS plan by epidemiological support POCs	–Demonstration of epidemiological support (data collection or analysis) in exercises, suspected CBR agent-related incidents, or natural disease outbreaks
–Evidence of interaction with and input to planning by POCs –Sign-off or other evidence of agreement with MMRS plan by laboratory support POCs	–Demonstration of laboratory support in exercises, CBR agent-related hoaxes, actual disaster, or CBR agent-related event
–Evidence of formal or informal agreements with organizations designated to provide emergency security personnel (e.g., National Guard, private security firms)	–Demonstration of availability of anticipated assets on short notice for random check, planned exercise, or actual emergency –Time from request to appearance on site if request is for immediate help –After-action reports from events with large attendance such as sporting events, concerts, and political conventions
–Same as 3.18	–Same as 3.18
–Meeting minutes or other evidence of exercise planning	–Evidence that exercises were completed on schedule –A collection of after-action reports
–Meeting minutes or other evidence of after-action report production, including revisions or comments by key agencies –Documented process for evaluation of exercises for development of after-action reports and addressing the recommendations of those reports	–Possession by all participating agencies and institutions of the collection of after-action reports –Evidence for changes in structure or functioning in response to reported deficiencies

Deliverable 3: Continued

Plan Elements	Inputs
3.22 Designation of mental health care for emergency workers, victims and their families, and others in community needing special assistance	–List of local mental health practitioners and sources of extralocal practitioners –SOPs for provision of on-scene and community support
3.23 Provisions for proper examination, care, and disposition of fatalities (see Plan elements 7.09, 7.10, and 7.11)	–List of facilities or sites for expanded operations of medical examiner or coroner –List of local undertakers –List of local religious leaders –Disaster Mortuary Operational Response Team (DMORT) POCs

Deliverable 4: MMRS Plan for Forward Movement of Patients Using the National Disaster Medical System (NDMS)

Plan Elements	Inputs
4.01 Detailed procedures for preparation of patients for movement to other areas of the region or nation	–A fully developed SOP
4.02 Identification of who makes the decision to implement forward movement of patients	–Name(s) of individual(s) at each patient care facility to make decision
4.03 Indication that NDMS would provide transportation and care	–Text of plan and NDMS POC –Signed agreements between participating hospitals and NDMS

Processes	Outputs
–Evidence of interaction with local mental health organization or agency –Agreements with private organizations and individual practitioners to provide mental health services for all segments of population –Evidence of practitioner training or experience providing services to disaster victims and/or responders	–After-action reports from other kinds of disasters or exercises that document coordination, availability, use, and effectiveness of mental health professionals
–Meeting minutes or other evidence of interaction with POCs in funeral business and religious community regarding mass fatalities –MOUs, contracts, or other evidence of support of MMRS plan by undertaking and religious POCs	–After-action reports from other disasters or crimes that document satisfactory processing of large numbers of human remains –Evidence of tabletop exercises testing disposition plans and procedures for fatalities

Processes	Outputs
–Distribution of SOPs to emergency medical services (EMSs), local hospitals	–Awareness of plan and SOPs by EMSs and hospital officials and when and how to initiate them
–Appointment or notification letter, instructions	–Sign-off by designated individual(s)
–Documentation of contact with NDMS –Identification of their own and federal POCs for facilities with signed NDMS agreements	–Evidence of NDMS support for MMRS plan and SOPs for activation (e.g., from joint training, tabletop demonstration of interface)

Deliverable 5: MMRS Plan for Chemical and Radiological Events

Plan Elements	Inputs
5.01 Procedures for effective management of the health consequences of a chemical or radiological incident	–Medical protocols for at least the chemical agents specified in the MMRS program contract (nerve agents, blister agents, choking agents, and blood agents) –Medical protocols for radiation injuries
5.02 Detailed procedures for detection and identification of agents	–Detectors for all agents specified in the MMRS program contract –SOPs for use of detectors –National Fire Prevention Association (NFPA) standards for hazmat operations
5.03 Detailed procedures for extraction of victims from incident site	–SOPs reflecting state laws and local regulations and practices –NFPA standards on extraction of victims
5.04 Detailed procedures for administration of appropriate antidote	–SOPs reflecting state laws and local regulations and practices –Medical protocols for all agents specified in contract
5.05 Detailed procedures for decontamination of victims	–SOPs reflecting state laws and local regulations and practices –List of any special equipment required
5.06 Procedures for victim triage and initial care before transport to definitive medical care facility	–SOPs reflecting state laws and local regulations and practices

Processes	Outputs
–Distribution of copies to all relevant sites –Percentage of medical personnel trained to deal with chemical and radiological agents –Number of classes conducted –Training schedule –List of trained medical personnel and date of training	–Hands-on demonstration (for peer reviewer or in a large-scale drill or actual hazmat incident) of knowledge of the protocol –Certification or other nationally recognized affirmation of CBR agent-specific knowledge and skills, if such means of verification become available in the future
–Percentage of hazmat personnel trained to deal with chemical and radiological agents –Number of classes conducted –Training schedule –Training log	–Hands-on demonstration (for peer reviewer or in a large-scale drill or actual hazmat incident) of agent detection and identification
–Percentage of rescue personnel trained to deal with chemical and radiological agents –Number of classes conducted –Training schedule –Training log	–Hands-on demonstration (for peer reviewer or in a large-scale drill or actual hazmat incident) of safe and efficient extraction of a victim from a contaminated area
–Percentage of eligible emergency medical personnel trained to deal with chemical and radiological agents –Number of classes conducted –Training schedule –Training log	–Hands-on demonstration (for peer reviewer or in a large-scale drill or actual hazmat incident) of administration of proper antidote
–Percentage of personnel trained to deal with chemical and radiological agents –Number of classes conducted –Training schedule –Training log	–Hands-on demonstration (for peer reviewer or in a large-scale drill or actual hazmat incident) of decontamination of victims –List of all required equipment on hand or readily accessible
–Number of classes conducted –Training schedule –Training log –Percentage of personnel trained	–Hands-on demonstration (for peer reviewer or in a large-scale drill or actual hazmat incident) of victim triage and initial care

Deliverable 5: Continued

Plan Elements	Inputs
5.07 Provisions for emergency medical transportation of victims	–Inventory of transport vehicles – SOPs reflecting state laws and local regulations and practices –Current contracts and local procedures
5.08 Provisions for emergency and inpatient services in hospitals with capacity and capability for definitive care required or at designated off-site treatment facilities (1,000 victims of chemical agent release)	–List of hospitals, with the identification of capability of each to provide definitive care in individual clinical specialties –List of potential off-site treatment facilities –Designated individual to decide on need and location of off-site facilities –Poison Control Center staff contact information
5.09 Procedures for management of patients arriving at hospitals without prior field screening or decontamination	–Shower or other source of running water –Provisions for maintaining privacy of patients during decontamination –Personal protective equipment for staff –Source of heat in cold weather –Procedure for securing personal valuables of victims –Written procedures available to emergency department (ED) personnel –Procedure for rapidly establishing medical records for arriving patients
5.10 Procedures for procurement and provision of appropriate pharmaceuticals for up to 1,000 victims (see Deliverable 10)	–List of antidotes and pharmaceutical equipment and supplies appropriate for the designated agents –Purchase plan for appropriate antidotes and drugs –Written procedures for maintenance, disposition, deployment, and resupply
5.11 Procedures for procurement and provision of appropriate equipment and supplies (see Deliverable 10)	–List of equipment and supplies appropriate for the designated agents, considering the needs of both adult and pediatric patients –Purchase plan for appropriate equipment and supplies –Written procedures for maintenance, disposition, deployment, and resupply –List of suppliers with additional critical materials

Processes	Outputs
–MOUs and other agreements with private and public entities for emergency transport (buses, vans, trucks)	–Demonstration of availability of vehicles and response times in exercises or actual mass-casualty events
–MOUs or other acknowledgment of MMRS plan by listed hospitals and sites	–Expert opinion on adequacy of response in exercise or actual mass-casualty event
–Evidence of training –Evaluation by Joint Commission for Accreditation of Healthcare Organizations	–Actual decontamination of individual patients in small CBR agent-related or other hazmat incidents –Successful decontamination of multiple patients in an exercise or actual hazmat event
–Periodic inventory (see Deliverable 10)	–Demonstration that appropriate types and quantities of antidotes and drugs are on hand or readily accessible –Demonstration of timely deployment of stocks in an exercise or actual event (see Deliverable 10)
–Periodic inventory, including checks that perishable supplies and pharmaceuticals are within their "use by" dates (see Deliverable 10)	–Demonstration that appropriate types and quantities of equipment and supplies are on hand or readily accessible –Demonstration of timely deployment of stocks in exercise or actual event (see Deliverable 10)

Deliverable 6: Component Plan for Metropolitan Medical Strike Team (MMST) if Community MMRS Includes Such a Team

Plan Elements	Inputs
6.01 MMST mission statement and concept of operations	–Text of plan, including mission and concept of operations
6.02 Organization and membership of the team	–Mission statement and concept of operations –Organizational chart
6.03 Detailed procedures for activation and deployment	–Development and distribution of SOPs
6.04 Detailed procedures for identification of agent	–See 5.02
6.05 Detailed procedures for extraction of victims from the incident site	–See 5.03
6.06 Detailed procedures for administration of appropriate antidote	–See 5.04
6.07 Detailed procedures for human decontamination	–See 5.05
6.08 Detailed provisions for triage and initial care of victims	–See 5.06
6.09 Detailed preparation of victims for transport to definitive care facilities with sufficient supplies of appropriate antidotes to ensure adequate treatment	–See 5.06 and 5.07

Processes	Outputs
	–Explanation of mission and concept of operations to peer reviewer by representatives of key MMRS program institutions
–Organizational chart and current list of names and contact information for membership of the team	–Description of organization and membership of the team to peer reviewer by selected sample of team members –Inclusion of all necessary areas of expertise on the team
–Regular testing of activation procedures –Periodic testing of deployment SOPs	–Evidence of speed and completeness of activation and deployment in exercises or actual incidents
–See 5.02	–See 5.02
–See 5.03	–See 5.03
–See 5.04	–See 5.04
–See 5.05	–See 5.05
–See 5.06	–See 5.06
–See 5.06 and 5.07	–See 5.06 and 5.07

Deliverable 7: MMRS Plan for Biological Agent Events

Plan Elements	Inputs
7.01 Integration with existing local and state health surveillance plans for bioterrorism and influenza pandemic planning	–Relevant disease surveillance plan that includes regular and timely reporting from hospitals and independent medical doctors, as well as the capacity to analyze (in real time) trends and suspicious reports
7.02 Coverage of early recognition, mass immunization or prophylaxis, mass patient care, mass-fatality management, and environmental surety	–MMRS plan
7.03 Identification of early-warning indicators that will be used to alert local officials of a bioterrorism event	–List of plausible indicators (e.g., 911 calls, emergency medical service responses, poison control center calls, ED visits, medical examiner reports, school and work absenteeism, and reports from veterinarians of sick or dead animals) –Designated individual or office responsible for monitoring indicators –List of local officials to be notified of possible bioterrorism event (or outbreak of disease) –POCs for laboratory diagnosis system that includes field sampling, local laboratory screening, and public health laboratory network connection and capacity –List of trained personnel (and on-call schedules) to conduct epidemiological investigations and analyses to determine the scope and magnitude of the epidemic
7.04 Identification of who will receive notification and who will make the decision to further implement response plans	–Name, organization, and position of designated individual
7.05 New plans or augmentation of existing plans for management and implementation of a mass immunization or prophylaxis plan (also see Deliverable 10)	–MMRS plan or augmented preexisting plan –Stockpile or plans for acquisition and storage of appropriate vaccines, antibiotics, and antitoxins –List of potential sites for mass immunization or prophylaxis –List of personnel or sources of personnel to conduct mass immunization or prophylaxis –List of personnel or sources of personnel to distribute vaccines or antibiotics to sites of mass immunization or prophylaxis –System for recording persons who have received mass immunization or prophylaxis

Processes	Outputs
–Evidence of regular communication among local, state, and federal public health entities (e.g., memos, MOUs, site surveys, software interaction) –Regularly maintained baseline data on reportable diseases	–Evidence of ongoing disease detection from actual cases, interviews by peer reviewers, or exercises or tests –Demonstration of effective surveillance for specific events (mass gatherings, controversial trials, etc.)
–None required	–MMRS plan that addresses early recognition, mass immunization or prophylaxis, mass patient care, mass-fatality management, and environmental surety
–Daily records or charts of baseline data from indicator collection system – Established thresholds above which action is required –Record of training for laboratory personnel on assays for detection of agents responsible for the diseases specified in the contract (anthrax, botulism, hemorrhagic fevers, plague, smallpox, and tularemia) –Record or schedule of laboratory quality assurance training and testing	–Demonstration of appropriate use of early-warning indicators in peer-review interview, exercise, or actual event –Percentage of laboratory personnel certified by relevant professional organization –Demonstration to peer reviewer of knowledge and availability of supplies to carry out specified assays or successful detection of a test sample containing a close relative of one of the designated agents
–Evidence that the office monitoring indicators knows the name of designated individual and has multiple means of relaying relevant information	–Confirmation by designated individual that he or she is the appropriate contact and demonstration that he or she is conversant with the MMRS plan
–Percentage of response and caregiving personnel immunized if plan calls for prophylactic immunization of these individuals –MOUs or other evidence that sites and designated personnel are aware of and knowledgeable about their roles in the plan –See Deliverable 10 for preparedness indicators for supplies and equipment	–After-action report detailing successful response to a natural outbreak of disease (e.g., a meningitis or influenza vaccine campaign) or large-scale exercise

Deliverable 7: Continued

Plan Elements	Inputs
7.06 Description of the decision-making process for initiating a mass immunization campaign and identifying the affected population	–MMRS plan that designates an individual (name, organization, and position) to make the decision to provide immunization or prophylaxis to staff and the community and the criteria to be used –Legal and regulatory references that provide the designated individual with the requisite authority
7.07 New plans or augmentation of existing plan for providing care to a significant portion of the population (see Plan Element 7.08 and Deliverables 6 and 8)	–Comprehensive list of facilities, with POCs and telephone and fax numbers –Number of beds, isolation capacity, and infection control capacity in the community, including special centers for care –Mass-casualty plans of area hospitals –Medical protocols for at least the agents specified in the MMRS program contract (those responsible for anthrax, botulism, hemorrhagic fever, plague, smallpox, and tularemia)
7.08 Detailed procedures for rapid expansion of the existing health care system capacity and plans for taking care of people in excess of either existing or expanded capacity (see Deliverables 6 and 8)	–Number of beds, isolation capacity, and infection control capacity in the community, including special centers for care –Mass-casualty plans of area hospitals –List of medical personnel not employed full time by area hospitals or sources of such personnel –List of potential sites for expedient patient care facilities, with the rationale for their selection
7.09 New plans or augmentation of existing mass-fatality plans for respectful care and disposition of a large percentage of the population	–Existing plan –MMRS plan
7.10 Procedures for augmentation of existing morgue facilities and staff	–List of hospital morgues, mortuaries, warehouses, other facilities with cold-storage capabilities, and sources of refrigerated trucks, with POCs –Contact information for federal support via specialized DMORT

Processes	Outputs
–Verification that designated individual is cognizant of designation, legal authority, and SOPs –MOUs or other evidence of agreement by all parties to the plan	–After-action report detailing successful response to a natural outbreak of disease (e.g., a meningitis or influenza vaccine campaign) or large-scale exercise
–Evidence of periodic updates of information on beds and other resources –MOUs or other evidence of coordination by hospitals to make optimal use of available personnel, supplies, and equipment –Annual exercise of mass-casualty plans –Distribution of copies of medical protocols to all relevant sites	–Remedy of deficiencies identified by after-action reports of mass-casualty exercises –Hands-on demonstration (in response to peer reviewer questions or in a drill or actual disease outbreak) of interhospital coordination of personnel, equipment, and supplies –Hands-on demonstration (in response to peer reviewer questions or in a drill or actual disease outbreak) of treatment protocol knowledge by medical personnel
–MOUs or other agreements with participating agencies, institutions, and organizations –Contingency contracts for use of nonmedical sites for casualty collection and expedient patient care	–Hands-on demonstration (in a drill or actual disease outbreak) of ability to rapidly expand health care system capacity
–See 7.10 and 7.11	–See 7.10 and 7.11
–Contingency contracts or other forward arrangements for obtaining storage capacity –Evidence of NDMS support for MMRS plan and SOPs for activation (joint training, tabletop demonstration of interface with DMORT)	–No-notice test of system to determine if surge assets could be made available

Deliverable 7: Continued

Plan Elements	Inputs
7.11 Procedures for decontamination or isolation of human remains when appropriate	–SOPs covering decision to decontaminate and the decontamination process
7.12 Procedures for identification of environmental risk and determination of the need for decontamination or vector intervention	–List of local, state, and federal environmental agencies, with POCs –Detection and agent identification equipment capable of verifying safety –Mass medical and infectious waste management plans
7.13 A process for safe reentry into the affected area in consultation with local, state, and federal environmental agencies	–List of local, state, and federal environmental agencies, with POCs –Detection and agent identification equipment capable of verifying safety
7.14 Three levels of response: for incidents with up to 100 victims, 100 to 10,000 victims, and more than 10,000 victims **IOM Alternative** Three capacity levels: normal capacity, capacity with augmentation, and "overwhelmed" level	–Evaluation of each of the Deliverable 7 inputs described above relative to each of the three scenarios

Processes	Outputs
–Evidence that SOPs are available at morgue facilities in sufficient quantity to distribute to any expedient sites and personnel required	–Hands-on demonstration of decontamination in an exercise or actual incident
–See 7.13	–See 7.13
–Record of agreement with the MMRS plan by local, state, and federal environmental agencies –Awareness by the individual or agency charged with judging safety of responsibility and has SOP for decision making	–Demonstration of an effective process to expert peer reviewer; in response to questioning; or by performance in an exercise, actual hazmat event, or disease outbreak
–Evaluation of each of the Deliverable 7 processes described above relative to each of the three scenarios	–Evaluation of each of the Deliverable 7 outputs described above relative to each of the three scenarios

Deliverable 8: MMRS Hospital Plan

Plan Elements	Inputs
8.01 Procedures for notification of hospitals, clinics, health maintenance organizations (HMOs), etc., that an incident has occurred	–Comprehensive list of facilities, with POCs and telephone and fax numbers –Designated individual or office to initiate process, staff to carry it out –Communications equipment appropriate for rapid notice, e.g., radio, broadcast fax, or e-mail
8.02 Procedures for protection of hospitals, clinics, and HMOs from contamination from environmental or patient sources (lockdown procedures)	–Presence of plan at all local health care facilities –Availability of personal protective equipment required by plan –Capacities of facilities to secure all entrances and exits
8.03 Provisions for the capability of local health care facilities to provide triage and initiate definitive care	–Inventory of services and capabilities –Specification by each facility of three levels of capability: normal operations, operations with augmentation, and overwhelmed operations –SOPs on transfer process
8.04 Assurance of adequate security to support provision of emergency and definitive health care during and following a large-scale terrorism event	–MMRS plan –List of available law enforcement and security assets, with POCs

Processes	Outputs
–Periodic notification checks conducted at least weekly, including at nights, on weekends, and on holidays	–Percentage of facilities contacted in 1 hour during weekly notification checks –Time from initial contact to initiation of hospital disaster plan or incident command system –Time from initial contact until hospitals report beds and capabilities are available
–Evidence that personnel at all facilities are provided orientation on plan –Evidence that all facilities have SOPs and provide training to staff on safe care of highly infectious patients (e.g., patients with varicella, tuberculosis, or drug-resistant infections)	–Numbers of secondary infections of staff or other patients in prior 6 months –Current conversion rate for positivity for tuberculosis (purified protein derivative) skin tests among staff –Numbers of isolation rooms available, overall and in the ED –Numbers of tuberculosis, rubella, or varicella patients admitted to nonisolation rooms in prior 6 months –Numbers of staff furloughed due to exposure to patients with varicella, rubella, or other infectious diseases in prior 6 months –Numbers of hours from examination of most recent tuberculosis patient to isolation
–Evidence that facilities have clear policies and procedures for handling of ED overload and ED diversion	–Numbers, types, and durations of diversions in previous 3 months –Numbers and types of patients transferred out of the hospital to other facilities in previous 3 months –Expert assessment of MMRS program-wide hospital exercise or response to mass-casualty event
–Evidence of formal or informal agreements with organizations designated to provide emergency security personnel (e.g., National Guard, private security firms) –Evidence that agreements include preexisting plans to allocate security staff when demand exceeds supply	–Anticipated assets available on short notice for a random check, planned exercise, or actual emergency –Number of unauthorized entrants during a drill or exercise

Deliverable 8: Continued

Plan Elements	Inputs
8.05 Availability of adequate personal protective equipment for hospital and clinic providers (see Deliverable 10)	–List of equipment needs –Purchase plan –Training plan for equipment users
8.06 Local availability of adequate pharmaceuticals and equipment (including ventilators) or plans to obtain them in a timely manner (see Deliverable 10)	–List of desired pharmaceuticals –Medical treatment protocols for agents specified in the fiscal year (FY) 2000 MMRS program contract (nerve agents; blister agents; choking agents; blood agents; and those responsible for anthrax, botulism, hemorrhagic fever, plague, smallpox, and tularemia) –Data on populations of communities participating in the MMRS program
8.07 Ability of medical staff to recognize and treat casualties caused by agents used as weapons of mass destruction (see 8.08)	–Communitywide list of physicians with hospital privileges, with telephone contact information –Medical treatment protocols for agents specified in MMRS program contract (nerve agents; blister agents; choking agents; blood agents; and those responsible for anthrax, botulism, hemorrhagic fever, plague, smallpox, and tularemia) in FY 2000 –Essential antidotes, antibiotics, and immune sera, in appropriate quantities
8.08 Availability of treatment protocols	–Medical protocols for at least the agents specified in the MMRS program contract (nerve agents; blister agents; choking agents; blood agents; and those responsible for anthrax, botulism, hemorrhagic fever, plague, smallpox, and tularemia)

Processes	Outputs
–Inventory of available equipment –Training logs	–Demonstration of competency with equipment (e.g., by a respirator fit test) for expert peer reviewer
–MOUs or other collaborative agreements with other local medical care facilities for emergency loan and distribution of required equipment and pharmaceuticals, including pediatric ventilators –SOPs for requesting CBR agent-specific equipment, supplies, and pharmaceuticals from MMRS program stores	–Availability of all essential antidotes, antibiotics, and immune sera, in appropriate quantities, for inspection by site-visit team or peer reviewer –Evidence of effective collaboration in coping with recent national shortages of influenza and tetanus vaccines and gamma globulin and emergency shortages of antibiotics –Response times required to retrieve requested items in drills or in actual cases
–Credentialing, where applicable –Continuing medical education (CME) roster or training schedule –Numbers and percentages of staff trained on protocols –Linkage to local, state, federal experts via telephone, e-mail, Health Alert Network, Internet, mass paging and alert systems, etc.	–Laboratory quality assurance test results –Demonstration of knowledge in responses to peer reviewer questions, exercise, or actual event –Certification or other nationally recognized affirmation of CBR agent-specific knowledge and skills, if such means for certification become available in the future –Number of hours from time of examination of tuberculosis patients to isolation –Number of isolation rooms available in ED and in total –Number of tuberculosis patients admitted to nonisolation rooms –Number of staff furloughed due to exposure to patients with varicella, rubella, or other infectious diseases
–Distribution of protocols to all physicians and availability of protocols at all major medical care sites –Training schedule –Numbers and percentages of staff trained on protocols	–Demonstration of knowledge by EDs, intensive care units, and primary care physicians and nurses in responses to peer reviewer questions, exercise, or actual event –Certification or other nationally recognized affirmation of CBR agent-specific knowledge and skills, if such means for certification become available in the future –Compliance with existing protocols

Deliverable 8: Continued

Plan Elements	Inputs
8.New 1. Procedures for recall of staff	–Telephone call list –Public communication plan –List of news media outlets and POCs
8.New 2. Procedures for delivery of nonmedical supplies (see Deliverable 10)	–List of customary and alternative vendors of food, fuel, laundry, and other essential supplies

Deliverable 9: MMRS Training Plan

9.01 Training requirements for all personnel responding to the scene of an incident or providing care to victims of a CBR agent-related incident	–Numbers and locations of police and fire department personnel, emergency medical technicians, paramedics, vehicle drivers, ED staff (physicians and nurses), hospital administration and infection control officers, chemical and radiation safety officers, local and regional public health authorities, and U.S. Department of Veterans Affairs (VA) hospital staff (if present in the community) –Numbers of qualified, trained instructors –Curricula consistent with prior discipline-specific training or training agreements with appropriate agencies –Hands-on as well as didactic training schedule –List of CBR agents addressed –Estimate of logistical support required
9.02 Indication of how training previously received from the U.S Department of Defense (DOD) or the U.S. Department of Justice (DOJ) affects initial training requirements, continuing education, and refresher training needs	–List of prior training conducted

Processes	Outputs
–Periodic tests of accuracy of phone numbers –Periodic tests of recall effectiveness –Test of recall lists to see how many facilities are counting the same people on recall list	–Evidence from calls to random sample of list shows that the list is up to date –Percentage of staff returning in 2 hours
–Contingency contracts with alternative suppliers –Periodic shortages drill	–Evidence of no disruption of services due to shortages during a drill or mass-casualty event –Response times for deliveries –Alternative supplier can deliver necessary supplies in 24 hours
–Numbers and contents of courses provided, both lecture and hands-on courses (e.g., disaster drills), with critiques provided to participants –Number of people (and percentage of the target workforce) trained –Number of communitywide exercises including disaster drills and tabletop exercises	–Demonstration of knowledge of subject matter to peer reviewer by selected sample of trained personnel from all levels of all participating organizations or through functional drills, communitywide exercises, or responses to actual CBR agent, hazmat, or infectious disease outbreak events –Certification or other nationally recognized affirmation of CBR agent-specific knowledge and skills, if such means for certification become available in the future
–Revision of training requirements reflecting previous training	

Deliverable 9: Continued

Plan Elements	Inputs
9.03 Description of VA's role in training medical personnel in NDMS hospitals	–Location of and POCs at nearest VA hospital –Agreement with VA hospital to provide training to non-VA employees on space-available basis –Numbers of qualified, trained instructors –Curricula consistent with prior discipline-specific training or training agreements with appropriate agencies –Hands-on as well as didactic training schedule –List of CBR agents addressed

Deliverable 10: MMRS Plan for Pharmaceuticals and Equipment

Plan Elements	Inputs
10.01 List of pharmaceuticals consistent with mission of MMRS program	–List of desired pharmaceuticals –MMRS program mission statement –Medical treatment protocols for agents specified in MMRS program contract (nerve agents; blister agents; choking agents; blood agents; and those responsible for anthrax, botulism, hemorrhagic fever, plague, smallpox, and tularemia) in FY 2000
10.02 Quantities of pharmaceuticals sufficient to care for 1,000 victims of a chemical agent and for entire affected population for 24 hours after a biological incident	–List of desired pharmaceuticals –Medical treatment protocols for agents specified in MMRS program contract (nerve agents; blister agents; choking agents; blood agents; and those responsible for anthrax, botulism, hemorrhagic fever, plague, smallpox, and tularemia) in FY 2000 –Data on populations of communities participating in the MMRS program
10.03 Timetable for procurement of pharmaceuticals and equipment	–Timetable for initial procurement and replenishment based on differences in essential pharmaceuticals, equipment, and personnel and those actually required in plan

Processes	Outputs
–Numbers and contents of courses provided, both lecture and hands-on courses (e.g., disaster drills), with critiques provided to participants –Number of people (and percentage of the target workforce) trained	–Demonstration of knowledge of subject matter to peer reviewer by selected sample of trained personnel

Processes	Outputs
–Periodic assessment of appropriateness of agents (outdating, currency of pharmacopoeia, changes in threat) by a pharmacy and therapeutics committee	–List that includes all treatments and vaccines specified in MMRS program medical treatment protocols
–Algorithm for calculating required quantities of pharmaceuticals –Verification that a project manager can explain the derivation of the algorithm to the satisfaction of an expert peer reviewer	–Availability of all essential antidotes, antibiotics, and immune sera, in appropriate quantities, for inspection by site-visit team or peer reviewer
–Establishment of mechanisms for review and update of pharmacopoeia –Establishment of mechanisms for monitoring pharmaceutical expiration dates and replacing stock	–Availability of all essential antidotes, antibiotics, and immune sera, in appropriate quantities, for inspection by site-visit team or peer reviewer

Deliverable 10: Continued

Plan Elements	Inputs
10.04 Detailed procedures for equipment maintenance and pharmaceutical storage	–Pharmacopoeia, with associated storage requirements –Equipment list, with associated maintenance requirements –Property officer(s) –SOPs for equipment maintenance –SOPs for pharmaceutical storage –Identification of secure storage site(s)
10.05 Identification of a property officer responsible for all property received and purchased under MMRS program contract	–Name and contact information for designated property officer
10.06 Harmonization of equipment purchases with equipment received from DOD, DOJ, and the Federal Emergency Management Agency	–List of essential detection, protective, and decontamination equipment for use both in the field and in hospitals –List of protective, detection, and decontamination equipment previously received from other federal sources
10.New 1 Procedures for distributing pharmaceuticals and equipment to local personnel and facilities	–List of authorized local recipients –SOPs for release of pharmaceuticals and equipment
10.New 2 Procedures for requesting, receiving, and distributing pharmaceuticals from the National Pharmaceutical Stockpile (NPS)	–SOPs, including phone and e-mail contacts at the Centers for Disease Control and Prevention (CDC) –Source of personnel for breaking down and distributing CDC "push package" to health care facilities –Licenses and approvals as required by federal, state, and local laws governing dispensing of pharmaceuticals

Processes	Outputs
–Periodic assessment of safety of storage and delivery systems –Periodic testing of appropriateness of drugs supplies (outdated supplies, currency of pharmacopoeia) by a pharmacy and therapeutics committee –Periodic drills, actual events, or questioning by expert peer reviewer demonstrate mechanisms for coordination of activity at multiple sites as well as return and decontamination of equipment and unused supplies –Records of periodic maintenance of equipment –Records of training of logistics personnel on maintenance procedures	–Evidence that the mechanism of delivery and storage is secure in natural disasters, mock drills, earthquakes, or hazmat events –Consistency of inventory with records of pharmacy and therapeutics committee meetings –Knowledge of procedures for return of unused supplies and decontamination of equipment by logistics personnel –Evidence that a sample of equipment selected by peer reviewer is in working order –Performance of required maintenance and/or prompt retrieval of maintenance manual by logistics personnel when queried by peer reviewer
–Records of purchase and current location of all property	–Retrieval of inventory and maintenance records by property officer –Evidence that a sample of property in acceptable condition can be produced for expert peer reviewer at locations specified in property officer records
–Purchase plan that reflects equipment and supplies on hand from other sources	–Evidence that sum of equipment on hand, on order, or scheduled for purchase is not greater than documented need
–Periodic training and testing of distribution plan	–Evidence from drill, actual event, or questioning by expert peer reviewer that local distribution of MMRS program pharmaceuticals and equipment will be rapid enough to maintain local supplies for at least the initial 24 hours of an event
–Periodic training and testing of distribution plan	–Evidence from drill, actual event, or questioning by expert peer reviewer that local distribution of NPS supplies will be rapid enough to maintain local supplies after the initial 24 hours of an event

F

Scenarios and Discussion Materials for Use on Site Visits

BIOLOGICAL SCENARIO (ANTHRAX)

Potential Participants

Fire department
Police department or sheriff's office
Office of Emergency Services
Public works department
Public health department
Public information officer
General counsel's office
Medical examiner or Coroner's Office
Emergency department physician
Transportation authority (port authority, airport authority, etc.)
Coordinator of volunteer organizations
Emergency medical service
Hazardous materials team
State emergency management office
Area military and local federal facilities
National Guard
U.S. Department of Energy
Federal Bureau of Investigation
Public Health Service
Centers for Disease Control and Prevention
Environmental Protection Agency

U.S. Coast Guard
Representatives of neighboring jurisdictions

The list is not intended to be either prescriptive or inclusive.

Instructor's Background Information on the Incident, Scene I

This scenario involving terrorism with a biological weapon of mass destruction (WMD) portrays an incident that local response groups and agencies can use to evaluate their coordination and response capabilities. They may also identify shortfalls in personnel or other resources that can be supplemented by state or federal sources. The scenario is intended to portray only the hypothetical technical features of a biological terrorism incident and does not represent an actual event.

This scenario takes place in [*city, state*]. [*Briefly describe the airport at which this incident occurs.*] In this scenario, a terrorist obtains four aerosol containers (emitting particles 1 to 5 micrometers in diameter); each is filled with 25 grams of freeze-dried, genetically altered *Bacillus anthracis* (anthrax) spores. The aerosol containers are placed in air ducts near baggage claim and ticketing areas within the airport, but immediately after the placement of the containers a security guard comes upon the terrorists and is stabbed.

Anthrax spores are biological agents that enter the body through inhalation, the primary danger in this scenario. Exposure to anthrax spores can also occur via breaks in the skin (open wounds, sores, and even very minor scratches). *B. anthracis* is a persistent agent capable of surviving in spore form for 1 to 2 years in direct sunlight or for decades if it is protected from direct sunlight.

The effects after an exposure normally appear within 2 to 3 days, although new cases occurred up to 60 days after a now well-characterized aerosol emission in Sverdlosk, Russia, in 1979. The initial symptoms of exposure to anthrax spores are low-grade fever and aches and pains, resembling the early stages of the flu. The illness progresses over 2 to 3 days until the sudden development of severe respiratory distress, followed by shock and death within 24 to 36 hours in essentially all untreated cases. The rate of mortality is high even with intensive supportive therapy and antibiotics, especially if treatment is delayed after the victim first exhibits symptoms.

An easily observable event indicating the initial release of anthrax spores is not necessary, and most planning has assumed that bioterrorism involving anthrax would be a covert release that would result in the wide dispersal of victims, both geographically and, because of varying incubation times, temporally. The only experience to date, however, has been with anthrax spore-contaminated letters in which the letters explicitly described their contents (in addition, hundreds of similar letters that falsely claimed to contain anthrax spores were also sent). In this scenario terrorists are nearly caught in the act, but it is not immediately clear that they are terrorists or that anthrax is involved. Indications of infection at its early stages can be confused with the symptoms that result from a wide variety of viral, bacterial, and fungal infections. Anthrax is therefore not immediately diagnosed.

Anthrax is difficult to detect through routine blood testing and culture when the agent is not suspected. Once a biological agent or anthrax is suspected, however, anthrax is easy to detect through more specific testing. There are several tests specifically for anthrax. Most of these require cultures, which can take 12 to 24 hours to produce results.

In this scenario it is not apparent at first that a biological agent was used. No terrorist organization called in a threat or claimed responsibility for the act. In fact, it is not until Scene II that terrorism emerges as the cause of this incident.

The medics responding to the stabbing in the airport do not suspect a terrorist attack and do not wear personal protective equipment. Anthrax spores contaminate the hospital where the initial victims are taken for treatment. People passing through the airport or coming into contact with any of these people are also potentially exposed. The [*area*] emergency medical services and police personnel responding to the stabbing are exposed as well.

Responders are challenged to

- assess the incident,
- initiate appropriate public health operations, and
- arrange for fast medical treatment of victims.

At this time, the local and state health departments and the Centers for Disease Control and Prevention (CDC) are involved in the community health emergency (prompted by notification by doctors and hospitals in the scenario) and the Emergency Operations Center (EOC) is activated. Many command and control issues are raised because this is initially treated as a community health emergency. These issues should be explored in Session I. The integration of federal assets should be discussed briefly during Session I, but it should also be discussed in further detail during Sessions II and III. It is not readily apparent that this is a terrorism-related incident. Once this is determined, during Scene II, notification of the Federal Bureau of Investigation (FBI) is required. The facilitator should explore how this notification takes place.

Scene I: The WMD Event Occurs

[*City, state, of the incident in the scenario*], [*day of week, date of the incident in the scenario*]. The weather forecast predicts [*insert the weather forecast for the scenario within the normal range for the date of the exercise; include the daily temperature range, the amount of cloud cover, and the wind speed and direction; if possible, set up the scenario for a calm, cool, overcast day*]. At midday it is [*temperature, in degrees Fahrenheit, within the forecasted range*].

On [*date of the exercise or the incident in the scenario*], at approximately 8 a.m. (0800 hours), a security guard at the airport confronts two men in coveralls exiting a restricted portion of the baggage claim area and is stabbed by one of the men. The men then flee into the crowd. The guard manages to call airport security before he loses consciousness. Police respond to the scene and call an ambulance. Paramedics arrive within 6 minutes and begin treating the security guard. Police try to locate passengers who may have seen the fleeing men.

By 5 p.m. (1700 hours) on [*day, date of the 3rd day of the scenario*], a number of airport workers at [*name of airport*] have reported to the occupational health clinic complaining of flulike symptoms. Throughout the following day, more and more workers complain of similar symptoms. The number of workers calling in sick or leaving work early due to illness increases dramatically. Affected workers visit numerous local doctors and hospitals.

By 3 p.m. (1500 hours) [*day, date of the 4th day of the scenario*], more than[*number equal to approximately 35 percent of the total number of airport personnel*] airport personnel call in sick, complaining of malaise, low-grade fever, and chest pains. The number of illnesses causes concern among airport operators about the ability of the remaining personnel to continue normal operations. The airport personnel office notes that many of the ill employees work in and around the ticketing and baggage claim areas. Doctors and hospitals notify the local health department, prompted by indications that the illness is reaching epidemic proportions. The state health department and the CDC in Atlanta, Georgia, are also notified.

The local news media picks up the story and broadcasts it locally. Other major cities across the nation, especially [*names of two of the major destinations from airport*], report scattered incidents of similar illnesses. Approximately half of the students and faculty at a school adjacent to the airport are also ill with flulike symptoms. Some visit local doctors and hospitals.

By [*day, date of the 5th day of the scenario*] at 9 a.m. (0900 hours), local hospitals report that approximately 30 airport workers are dead or critically ill; these deaths are reported to the [*name of state health department*] and the CDC. Another 2,000 individuals (former passengers) demonstrate flulike symptoms and visit doctors and hospitals throughout the metropolitan area; several have died. These illnesses are also reported to the [*name of state health department*] and the CDC. The CDC deploys an epidemiological research team to [*location of incident*] to assist the local and state health authorities as they continue their investigation and analysis.

The State Health Department notifies the [*name of state*] Emergency Management Agency (EMA) of the unfolding situation. The [*name of state*] EMA, in turn, notifies the regional office of the Federal Emergency Management Agency (FEMA) and the FBI. The Regional Operations Center (ROC), situated in [*location of ROC*], is activated.

The CDC investigation centers on the airport because it is a common denominator among the illnesses and deaths. Because of the number of sick and dead victims, the CDC and state health authorities recommend that the city shut down the airport until the site is thoroughly evaluated for health risks. The airport is shut down completely; outgoing flights are canceled and incoming flights are diverted to other regional airports. Health department personnel attempt to develop a strategy to track passengers and contact the families of passengers who may be infected; the CDC recommends that response personnel track all passengers who have passed through airport facilities in the past week. All personnel entering the airport after the shutdown order are issued biohazard protective gear that they must wear. Specimens are collected from hundreds of surfaces at the airport and sent to [*names of two nearest major hospitals or medical centers*].

Shortly after 10 a.m. (1000 hours) on [*day, date of the 6th day of the scenario*], epidemiological investigation reports released by the CDC suggest that a biological weapons agent may be the cause of the rash of illnesses and deaths.

By midday, the incident gains national media attention. The public inundates the airport and local hospitals with phone calls concerning potential contamination.

Reporters request information regarding the shutdown of the airport, its surrounding area, and the city's response to the incident. A major national cable news network requests an interview with a representative from the city. A Joint Information Center is established in the ROC to ensure that the CDC and state and local health departments as well as the FBI and state and local law enforcement agencies deliver accurate and consistent messages.

Facilitated Discussion

Purpose

This guided group discussion is designed to help participants understand the types of issues that they will encounter and the conflicts across agencies and jurisdictions that can occur in coordinating, communicating, and responding to such an incident. It also gives participants an opportunity to assess their jurisdiction's ability to respond to such an incident.

Presentation

Guide a group discussion by asking the numbered questions on the following pages. These questions are not all inclusive; use them to develop additional questions, as necessary. Some additional questions are included should there be a need to stimulate further discussion.

Don't forget that good facilitators speak much less than the participants. This is an assessment activity, not a formal instructional class.

Provide participants with a copy of the questions that does not include the answers to questions, additional questions, or the final note to the facilitator.

Be sure to touch on the following areas: direction and control, notification and activation, communications, warning and emergency public information, hazard assessment, and management of field response.

Questions, Scene I

1. How will you learn of this incident involving a WMD? What internal and external notifications should you make? Are you satisfied that the current notification process is timely and adequate? How does the delay in recognition of this event as an incident involving a WMD affect your procedures?

The emergency operations plan (EOP) of each jurisdiction and agency should contain an outline of notification procedures. The EOP review completed by the facilitator during the development portion of this activity should provide adequate detail to support facilitated discussion. The following provides general guidance.

In many jurisdictions, the 911 dispatcher serves as the hub of the notification system and notifies certain agencies or certain individuals, or both. In the case of anthrax and other biological agents with delayed effects, the activation and notification process would be more deliberate than normal. In many cases the EOC will become progressively staffed as the incident matures. By the time the event is recognized as an incident involving a WMD, most of the staff may be on site.

In most jurisdictions, the police and fire departments have excellent internal notification systems; however, other participating agencies may not. Check this during the EOP review. During the discussion explore if or how the police and fire departments could assist other agencies.

Walk participants through each step of the notification and activation process for an incident with immediate effects, for example, an incident involving a large bomb or a chemical WMD. Let them estimate their time of arrival and where they will be reporting. Contrast that approach with the delays associated with knowing that a biological incident has occurred.

Follow-up Questions:

Does your jurisdiction have a policy that prevents full activation of the emergency management system when it is not needed? How does the slow-to-develop nature of this incident affect your procedures?

The screening process should be defined in local EOPs and often relies on the local office of emergency management or the EOC (if it is staffed 24 hours a day) to serve as the decision maker.

The slow-to-develop nature of this incident will affect the EOC activation procedures dramatically. Use the EOP review to gain additional insight into how this issue will likely be addressed.

Who handles notification of state and federal authorities? Will the National Response Center be notified in this scenario?

The responsibility for state and federal notifications should be clearly defined in the local plan. For an incident of this magnitude, once the terrorism link is established, the National Response Center should be notified.

Without indicators of widespread immediate effects, will an incident command system (or other management) structure be established? How will the incident commander be determined?

Explore with the participants when or what staffing level constitutes a management structure that is operational.

2. What information, equipment, and actions are required by your jurisdiction to conduct the initial assessment of the incident? How do you anticipate information to be distributed among responders?

Allow the group to brainstorm.

Items discussed should include the following:

–a method to determine the numbers and locations of all patients with signs and symptoms similar to those of the dead airport workers,

–a method to determine the source and identity of the infectious agent and the extent and area of contamination, and

–a method to determine the decontamination requirements.

The plan review should provide details on the method for sharing information with responders.

3. What immediate decisions related to protective actions that should be taken should the jurisdiction make? How will those decisions be implemented?

Decision making related to the protective actions that should be taken is a critical issue, and the participants should be allowed sufficient time to discuss the ramifications of their decisions. The issue of evacuation versus sheltering versus quarantine should be explored. The EOP should provide a framework for making such decisions. In the case of biological agents with delayed effects, the "cat is most likely already out of the bag." Sheltering is not a viable option at this point. The immediate area and adjacent buildings should be evacuated because of the risks associated with inhaling particles resuspended in the air. Those assisting with any evacuation must use at least simple respiratory protection, and an area at the collection center should be designated for medical screening of evacuees. There will most likely be tremendous political pressure, especially from adjacent jurisdictions, to quarantine anyone who could have been exposed to a suspected biological agent. This should be considered a viable option because the specific agent has not been identified at this point of the scenario. Revisit this issue during the next scene after anthrax has been identified, because anthrax is not normally considered contagious.

Allow participants to discuss the issues of decontamination and triage strategies.

Follow-up Questions:

Should the jurisdiction be concerned about the possibility of additional attacks?

This is always a possibility, and the group should discuss what changes they will have to make to manage additional incidents of either a terrorism event involving a WMD or more common emergencies (e.g., fires and auto accidents).

What medical facilities are victims or patients being sent to? What types of information should the emergency medical services units relay to the hospitals in the area to prepare them to receive patients potentially contaminated with an unknown hazardous material? Should any areas be quarantined?

These questions focus on the initial medical response. Allow the participants to discuss this topic, if they bring it up. If an examination of this topic is not initiated by the participants, it will be fully examined during the discussion associated with Scene II.

4. How will the incident site be secured to ensure that the crime scene is protected after such a significant time delay? What access and egress control procedures should be implemented?

The EOP should provide details on contamination control procedures and crime scene protection as part of its WMD annex, if it exists.

Allow the participants in the group to discuss their security procedures and how these relate to their overall response strategy.

Access and egress control procedures should be included in the hazardous materials (hazmat) portion of the local plan. Determine the group's understanding of the importance of this issue.

5. Is the current number of trained, qualified personnel within your jurisdiction sufficient to respond to this incident? If not, where will you seek support to bridge these deficiencies?

A review of the EOP should provide an indication of the number of trained and qualified personnel.

Mutual support agreements with other local governments and state agencies should be discussed at this point.

The state EOP should be activated. The group should discuss how activation of the state EOP will affect operations.

The National Strike Force, the U.S. Department of Defense, and the Public Health Service are among the federal agencies with expertise in this area.

6. Will the city or county EOC be adequate for coordinating the response to this incident? Will a separate command center that is physically close to the incident site be required? What resources are available for outfitting this command center?

This information should be extracted from the EOP. It is assumed that an incident command system will be used.

Follow-up Questions:

How long will it take to have an EOC activated and fully operational? What are the capabilities of the center? Are these capabilities adequate to respond to an incident of the magnitude presented here?

In this scenario, the command post should be at the local EOC, so the answer will depend on how long it will take to activate the EOC and staff it appropriately and on whether the local EOC is in the affected area. If so, the use of an alternate site should be discussed.

The capabilities of the local EOC and the alternate EOC should be apparent from the plan review.

Instructor's Background Information on the Incident, Scene II

It is now 8:00 a.m. (0800 hours) on [*day, date of the 6th day of the scenario*], approximately 120 hours after the initial release of anthrax spores into the air ducts at [*name of airport*] and approximately 64 hours after the first airport workers complained of illness. At this point, the FBI is called to respond to the suspected terrorist attack. President [*name of U.S. president*] has not issued a disaster declaration through the Stafford Act; hence, the Federal Response Plan is not activated. At 5:00 p.m. (1700 hours), the president issues a disaster declaration for the state. The FBI is already on scene, but FEMA is not. The FBI initiates the structure for crisis management and takes the lead in the criminal investigation. When FEMA arrives, the structure changes to reflect the need for FEMA to lead the federal consequence management effort under the Terrorism Annex of the Federal Response Plan. *Because the Terrorism Annex is a new addition to the Federal Response Plan, it is likely that participants in this exercise will not be familiar with the differences in these structures. Some additional guidance in these areas may be necessary.*

The presence of anthrax is first suspected 122 hours after spore release [*10:00 a.m. on day 6*], although it is not confirmed through laboratory testing until 136 hours after spore release. The persistence of anthrax spores creates major problems, as the spores can be spread to other locations via people or equipment contaminated at the original site of spore release.

Thousands of travelers are stranded because of the shutdown of the airport; international and domestic flights are rerouted to other airports, increasing air traffic and causing delays in those areas. Airports to which flights are diverted are: [*provide a list of regional and local airports to which traffic for the area could be diverted.*] Many passengers who were contaminated at the airport continued their travels to other parts of the country and the world. The instructor should insure that the participants consider the difficulties associated with decontaminating all these individuals, and consider the consequences of failing to do so.

The huge number of casualties in this scenario quickly exhausts the limited local supply of medicines such as broad-spectrum antibiotics. Triage may be conducted as part of an actual response effort; the emphasis is placed on saving as many lives as possible, which means that the worst-off individuals who are likely to die are lower in treatment priority than individuals who can clearly be saved. It is noteworthy, however, that experience with victims of the anthrax spore-laden letters of October 2001 suggests that inhalation anthrax is not uniformly fatal even when treatment begins after patients are symptomatic.

The vast majority of *B. anthracis* strains are sensitive in vitro to penicillin. Penicillin-resistant strains exist naturally; and it is not difficult to induce resistance to penicillin, tetracycline, erythromycin, and many other antibiotics through laboratory manipulation of organisms. All naturally occurring strains tested to date have been sensitive to erythromycin, chloramphenicol, gentamicin, and ciprofloxacin. In the absence of information concerning antibiotic sensitivity, at the earliest signs of disease treatment should be instituted with oral ciprofloxacin or intravenous doxycycline every 12 hours. Supportive therapy for shock, fluid volume deficit, and maintenance of adequacy of the airway may all be needed. In cases in which a biological weapons attack is suspected, prophylaxis with ciprofloxacin or doxycycline is recommended for any individuals likely to have been exposed.

Means of vehicular access to the airport area are crowded, and great confusion exists. Approximately [*provide the approximately number of people that travel through the airport each day*] travel through the airport each day, so a total of [*number per day times seven*] people traveled through the airport in the week before the shutdown was ordered. Once a biological weapon agent is suspected, the response to the scene changes dramatically. Decontamination needs to be performed for persons (and their personal belongings, e.g., clothing and baggage) who had been or who are inside the airport and its immediate vicinity, including passengers, airline and airport workers, and response personnel already on the scene. Self-contained breathing apparatuses (SCBAs) need to be procured and used, although a filtering mask may be sufficient (most fire departments carry SCBAs at all times, but it would be unlikely that they would have enough equipment to supply SCBAs to all those responding to this incident). Protective clothing needs to be procured and worn by both law enforcement and medical investigators. "Hot," "warm," and safe zones need to be defined.

Individuals thought to have been exposed should begin a 60-day course of antibiotic treatment; if clinical signs of anthrax occur, patients should be treated as described above, but they will need additional supportive care, almost certainly as inpatients. If the anthrax vaccine is not available, antibiotic treatment should be continued for an additional 40 days.

If the anthrax vaccine is available, patients should be offered the option of vaccination at this point as protection against the possibility of very late germinating spores. It is believed that individuals must be exposed to a series of six vaccinations over a period of 18 months before the vaccine can be fully effective, but limited data from studies with humans suggest that completion of the first three doses of the recommended six-dose primary series (at 0, 2, and 4 weeks) provides some protection against both the cutaneous and the inhalation forms of anthrax. Contraindications for use of the vaccine are sensitivity to vaccine components (formalin, alum, benzethonium chloride) and a history of clinical anthrax. Reactogenicity is mild to moderate and lasts for up to 72 hours (tenderness, erythema, edema, or pruritus). A smaller proportion of individuals (<1 percent) experience more severe local reactions (e.g., anaphylaxis, which precludes additional vaccination). The vaccine should be stored at refrigerator temperature (it should not be frozen).

Hospitals in the area that serve patients contaminated with anthrax are [*list the hospitals and medical centers with the capability of treating mass casualties*]. Hospitals outside the immediate area that serve as back up are [*list nearby regional medical facilities that could be used, especially any facilities that have mutual-support agreements with local facilities*].

The primary focus of this session should be the recognition that federal assistance, whether it is requested or not, is on the way. The scenario is designed to overwhelm the local and state response capabilities. The challenge is integrating the local response with federal and state interests. The criminal investigation, coordinated by the FBI, has the potential to conflict with the humanitarian aspects of the response. This conflict was demonstrated in the TWA Flight 800 incident: families wanted the priority placed on body recovery, thus slowing down the investigation.

The instructor should describe the transition from use of the incident command system initially established at the scene to use of a the larger unified command that encompasses all agencies. If the group's assumptions about how this works appear inaccurate, the instructor must provide the necessary corrections.

A host of federal agencies are potentially involved. Besides the CDC and the FBI, they include elements of the Environmental Protection Agency, the U.S. Department of Health and Human Services, the U.S. Department of Transportation , and the U.S. Department of Defense. Optimal use of the resources of these agencies is a challenge in a real incident. A very important nonfederal agency is the American Red Cross, which offers invaluable assistance in dealing with family notification and reunification issues, as well as assisting stranded travelers. The American Red Cross may have difficulties with volunteers (and contracted responders) because they refuse to service the area or victims for fear of becoming infected.

The resources most likely required from the state National Guard include transportation, communications, and security, as well as expertise and resources related to biological warfare.

Scene II: Chaos in the City

It is still [*day of week, date of the 6th day of the incident in the scenario*] in [*city, state, of the incident in the scenario*]. The temperature is currently [*mid-day temperature in degrees Fahrenheit forecast for the scenario*] with an expected high temperature for the day of [*high temperature in degrees Fahrenheit forecast for the scenario*].

It is [*date of 6th day*], at 8 a.m. (0800 hours). Hospitals and local clinics note that people complaining of flulike symptoms and others in more advanced stages of infection continue arriving at epidemic levels. Most have either passed through the airport or come into close contact with someone who has. An autopsy of one of the first victims reveals that respiratory arrest precipitated death. Greatly oversized mediastinal lymph nodes are consistent with the hypothesis of anthrax. The six initial victims taken to [*name of largest hospital in the area*] all died, and autopsies of these victims also report enlarged mediastinal lymph nodes and respiratory arrest as the cause of death. Because of the suspected use of anthrax spores, cultures for the biological agent are requested. Results from the cultures are not available for at least another 12 hours.

Suspicion of the presence of a biohazard causes local authorities to keep the airport closed. Local response agencies are overwhelmed with the numbers of potentially exposed persons demanding treatment, potentially infected rescue personnel, and an increase in media interest in the incident. The governor declares a state of emergency, and immediately requests a presidential disaster declaration.

At 4:45 p.m. (1645 hours) on the same day, the FBI arrives and takes charge of the criminal investigation. A CDC investigative team arrives and begins laboratory processing to confirm the state laboratory diagnosis of anthrax. The CDC has flown a "push package" of pharmaceuticals and medical supplies from the National Pharmaceutical Stockpile into a neighboring city, but distribution is slow and hospitals are running out of antibiotics.

Airport personnel estimate that between the time of the first reported incidents and the subsequent closure of the airport facilities [*develop estimates based upon actual average passenger rates at the airport*], [*estimated number*] passengers continued through the airport to other destinations and [*estimated number*] remained in the metropolitan area.

Reports regarding significant numbers of similar types of deaths from [*names of four largest metropolitan destinations from the airport site of the incident*] metropolitan areas are broadcast over a major national cable news network. It is anticipated that [*appropriate percent of total number*] of passengers and [*appropriate percent*] of airport workers may be infected with the agent.

The number of potentially infected residents of the metropolitan area is not known. However, the CDC estimates that thousands of deaths may be anticipated within the next 48 hours if anthrax is the causative agent. Airport officials conducting an investigation determine that most of the more seriously ill airport workers and those who were initially sick work in the check-in and baggage claim areas. The FBI sends an investigative team to each area in an attempt to locate the origin of the incident.

On the same day, at 5 p.m. (1700 hours), the U.S. president issues a disaster declaration through the Stafford Act, activating the Federal Response Plan. The FBI Joint Operations Center, as described in the Federal Response Plan Terrorism Annex, is established and the Domestic Emergency Support Team is dispatched to [*location of the incident*]. One of the National Emergency Response Teams is flown in from FEMA headquarters. All lead agencies for emergency support functions are notified to assemble their teams for deployment to the Disaster Field Office once it has been designated. The Disaster Field Office, which will have additional federal resources, should be fully staffed and equipped in approximately 24 hours.

Traffic congestion from the self-evacuation of some neighborhoods interferes with response operations. The American Red Cross reports a shortage of shelter volunteers. Most fear coming into contact with contaminated residents and becoming infected.

Hospitals, clinics, and doctors' offices in the area are overwhelmed with people who fear they may have been exposed to anthrax and are demanding prophylactic antibiotics.

On [*day, date of the 7th day of the scenario*], at 2 a.m. (0200 hours), laboratory analyses conducted by the CDC confirm that *B. anthracis* spores are the infectious agent causing the epidemic. The CDC notifies state and local response agencies. They also report that the quantities suggest intentional dispersion by a terrorist group. Information on the symptoms, decontamination procedures, and treatment for anthrax is disseminated to hospitals and to local, state, and federal response agencies as they arrive on the scene. Because of the vast number of infected people, the CDC and the state health department estimate that contamination of the airport began 5 to 7 days earlier.

Samples collected and sent to laboratories for testing indicate that a portion of the city near the airport is contaminated to some extent.

In a statement to the press, President [*name of the U.S. president*] condemns the vile act of terrorism and vows to apply the full force of the government to punish the culprits.

Questions, Scene II

1. Who is in charge of the incident site? How will your agency's actions be coordinated with the actions of other agencies? What conflicts could arise from the need to simultaneously conduct extensive criminal investigatory and response functions? What conflicts may be anticipated between the overlapping federal, state, and local jurisdictions?

Explore the federal definitions of crisis management and consequence management. At the federal level, the FBI has authority over the incident site and is responsible for crisis management. FEMA has federal authority for consequence management, but it must conform to the directions of the FBI to protect as much of the crime scene as possible while providing the needed rescue and relief to protect the population. The Public Health Service and the CDC both have significant roles in consequence management when they must respond to biological agents. It is anticipated that most jurisdictions will follow this delineation of responsibilities.

Determine who is in charge of the local response for both consequence and crisis management and explore the role of the health department.

Determine the command or management structure to be used by the jurisdiction. The Incident Command System has been adapted by many jurisdictions as their command structure during response operations. Explore the specifics of the local system during this discussion. A review of the EOP should have provided details on the structure of the command structure.

Conflicts will likely be related to the jurisdiction's attempt to balance protecting evidence and protecting people. Overlapping conflicts can occur as state and federal responders arrive on scene and the transition to a unified, joint, or coordinated command or management structure begins. During a health emergency the additional authority granted to the health department is also a source of potential conflict.

2. What community health planning has been completed? Have privately owned hospitals, home-care agencies, long-term-care facilities, and clinics been incorporated into the EOP and included in the planning process? Has your community conducted joint exercises for this type or any type of mass-casualty situation?

The EOP review should indicate the preparedness of the community health program to address mass-casualty situations and the involvement of all local health care assets in the planning process.

Most jurisdictions should have been involved in joint mass-casualty exercises because these are an accreditation requirement for most health care organizations, especially hospitals.

Follow-up Questions:

What community medical operations might be necessary?

This issue should be addressed in the community health plan as it exists. The priorities at the scene should be gross triage and screening at some type of collection or screening point. Transportation of potentially affected members of the population is another operational issue that should be addressed.

Will triage stations be established? Where will these be established?

The discussion of triage should focus on managing the flow of casualties through the community health system. The community health plan should address this issue.

Triage protocols at both collection and delivery points should also be part of the plan. Basic requirements dictate that triage be performed at both locations. This may be a good point to address the differences between standard emergency room triage and mass-casualty triage in most incidents involving a WMD. Contrast the immediate lifesaving needs associated with threats such as chemical agents and the more deliberate, supportive approach associated with biological agents.

What specific assistance do you need from the state and federal governments? How will these resources be integrated into the response operations?

State and federal plans provide for mobilization of these types of resources in disaster situations. It is important for the group to realize that there may be a significant time delay before those resources are available.

What type of epidemiological surveillance program does your community have in place? How well defined are the linkages between the community health program and plan and your consequence management infrastructure?

Epidemiological surveillance is important in determining the number of individuals who were exposed to the biological agent. Community health planning should account for locating within the incident area personnel who may be asymptomatic at this point, especially in light of the potential delayed and long-term health effects.

The community should consider establishing a database to track the health of those members of the community, including responders, who may have been exposed to anthrax.

The EOP should define the linkage between the community health program and the emergency operations management structure, and a representative of the community health agency or emergency medical services should be on the management team.

3. What immediate public relations and media concerns must be anticipated? How will these concerns be addressed? Who will serve as your jurisdiction's spokesperson in this incident?

The Joint Information Center should be established after the arrival of state and federal assets and should serve as the source of pubic information after that point. The plan should identify who will serve as the local spokesperson before the establishment of the Joint Information Center.

Most EOPs assign the management of public affairs issues to the management team located in the EOC. Determine participants' familiarity with public affairs procedures. Anticipating that public panic and extreme fear are likely to exist, the group should discuss how to diffuse the issue without denigrating the seriousness of the situation. Determine if the participants understand the importance of a multimedia approach and the development of themes.

Follow-up Question:

Does the communications system meet the multilingual needs of the area?

The EOP review should identify the multilingual needs of the community and procedures for meeting those needs.

4. What are the internal and external communications requirements for this response? Who is responsible for ensuring that the necessary systems are available? What problems may be anticipated?

The EOP should address internal and external communications requirements and assign responsibility for maintaining a viable system. Communications support equipment is normally located in or adjacent to the EOC.

Internal communications issues focus on the ability of jurisdictions to communicate with responders from different agencies (e.g., fire departments talking to police). Determine what system is in place to facilitate such coordination or if coordination must be accomplished face to face, through dispatchers, or through the EOC.

External communications issues should focus on the procedures for providing essential information to state and federal responders and managers who are en route to the incident site.

Solutions that rely on public hard telephone lines or cellular telephone systems should be discouraged in light of the numerous demands that will be made on those systems, unless the plan review revealed that a priority override system for emergency communications is in place with local telephone service providers.

Instructor's Background Information on the Incident, Scene III

It is now 8:00 a.m. on [*date of the 7th day of the scenario*], 6 full days after the release of anthrax spores at the airport. At this point, the FBI has effectively established control of the situation for crisis management purposes. The casualty figures could be horrendous. The potential for further spread of the spores exists, but levels of contamination beyond the airport and the surrounding neighborhoods may be so low that no further deaths may be reported due to the additional spread. The CDC is actively involved in supporting the community's consequence management effort, and adequate amounts of antibiotics are rushed to local treatment centers.

The response required all of the city's emergency response forces and most of those available from the county and other nearby cities. The stress and trauma of dealing with death on such a large scale affect many responders at the scene.

Crew relief schedules should be discussed in this session. Decontamination is expected to last many weeks, and no decision is made yet about airport operations.

The extended use of police and security forces can lead to problems in other areas of the city. In addition, the overload on the city's telephone system makes it nearly impossible to call anywhere in the area.

Scene III: The Immediate Threat Wanes

It is 9 p.m. (2100 hours) on [*day of week and date of 6th day of scenario*] in [*city, state, of the incident in the scenario*].

Additional medical supplies arrive on the scene and at local hospitals, including large quantities of ciprofloxacin and doxycycline.

Standard antibiotics are ineffectual in fighting anthrax infection among victims. Further studies conducted by the CDC indicate that the strain of anthrax used in the release may have been biologically manipulated to resist treatment and initiate symptoms much faster than normal. Hospitals seek additional information from the CDC as to what other courses of treatment may be used to combat anthrax infection.

The Disaster Field Office is established at [*location of Disaster Field Office*] and is fully staffed and equipped by the morning of [*7th day of the scenario*].

There are concerns about disposal of the victims' bodies. The number of victims and fear of spreading anthrax spores create problems with storage of the remains. The number of bodies collected overwhelms the city morgue and surrounding morgues. The total death count is more than 1,000. Hundreds of more deaths are anticipated. Families of the victims call local hospitals to arrange for retrieval of their loved ones' bodies for burial.

The CDC continues to collect samples from the areas downwind of the airport.

On the morning of [*date of the 8th day of the scenario*], at approximately 9 a.m. (0900 hours), airlines contact the CDC and the state health department with questions about testing for anthrax contamination on aircraft, equipment, and other potentially contaminated areas. They want to know what decontamination procedures will ensure the safety of their aircraft. Aircraft operators also ask if and when the airport will be safe to resume normal business.

The CDC and the state health department continue to generate detailed information on appropriate methods for the cleanup of contamination with anthrax spores. Information on long-term cleanup of the airport and affected areas indicates that thorough cleaning of the airport and surrounding areas must be completed before the areas can be reopened for normal business. President [*name of the U.S. president*] has already made it clear to the public that the airport will not reopen until laboratory testing confirms that it is free of contamination with anthrax spores.

Later that morning, FBI investigative teams locate the canisters used to spread the anthrax in the air ducts of the baggage claim and ticketing areas. There are no leads to the perpetrator(s) of the attack at this time. However, the FBI confirms that this incident is unquestionably a terrorism incident.

Media interest in the incident captures worldwide attention as the total victim count is confirmed. The incident sends shock waves through the country. People nationwide cancel flights and opt for alternate modes of transportation.

Representatives of the media transmit live interviews from the city reporting that residents are reluctant to return to their homes, despite assurances that it is safe to reenter designated areas.

Questions, Scene III

1. How will you conduct extended response operations? Are local personnel and equipment resources adequate for the extended operations required?

The EOP should account for round-the-clock operations. Many jurisdictions plan to send a portion of the EOC staff home after the initial incident assessment reveals the need for extended operations. Determine who will be responsible for each function on multiple shifts.

Each agency will likely be overwhelmed. The real question is how much state, federal, or National Guard support is needed.

2. What are your procedures for integrating state and federal resources into your management organization?

The EOP should outline the procedures for integration of state and federal resources.

State and federal assistance is supplementary to the local response; and as the Disaster Field Office is established, the Federal Coordinating Officer and State Coordinating Officer will coordinate the activities of the state and local governments, the American Red Cross, the Salvation Army, and other relief and disaster assistance organizations.

Follow-up Questions:

How will your agency coordinate its action with other agencies (federal, state, and local) and public interest groups?

The Federal Coordinating Officer is the primary federal coordinating authority for consequence management; the FBI handles crisis management.

With the arrival of state and federal assistance and the formation of a Joint Information Center, how will media inquiries be handled? Who in your jurisdiction is responsible for authoring media releases?

Media releases must be coordinated with the FBI, FEMA, and state and local authorities once the Federal Coordinating Officer has been established.

The EOP should provide a detailed communications and public relations plan.

3. What continuing assessments should be enacted when the cleanup phase is complete? Who will make these determinations?

Long-range health issues are of great concern.

The EOP should provide an overview of how continuing assessments and long-term monitoring are accomplished. Allow the participants in the group to discuss their areas of concern and to propose priorities.

4. What are the environmental concerns related to this incident?

Materials used during the response to support decontamination operations will continue to present hazards until they are neutralized.

Follow-up Questions:

What steps will be taken by your agency to ensure adequate sanitation measures throughout the affected area?

The local hazmat plan should identify sanitation procedures related to biological operations.

What local requirements exist for reentry to an evacuated area due to a biological agent incident?

The hazmat annex to the EOP should outline procedures for reentry into an evacuated area.

After the use of an especially persistent biological agent such as B. anthracis, *the local emergency management team should consider the need for "safe certification," that is, having a third-party laboratory verify that the area is free from contamination.*

5. Within your jurisdiction, what psychological traumas may be anticipated? How will your agency deal with these traumas?

Many agencies have teams already designated to assist in such cases. In most instances, the teams will not have the capacity to handle the expected number of cases in an incident of this magnitude.

Discuss the availability of crisis counseling. Also, refer participants to Section 416 of the Stafford Act.

Follow-up Questions:

How will your agency participate in notification of the deaths of civilians and your colleagues? Are personnel in your agency adequately trained in the process of death notification?

Death notification is always a difficult issue. The EOP should provide guidance to managers. However, at a minimum someone in the supervisory chain should be involved with the actual notification.

CHEMICAL SCENARIO (SARIN)

Potential Participants

Fire department
Police department or sheriff's office
Office of Emergency Services
Public works department
Public health department
Public information officer
General counsel's office
Medical examiner or coroner's office
Emergency department physician
Transportation authority (port authority, airport authority, etc.)
Coordinator of volunteer organizations
Emergency medical service
Hazardous materials team
State emergency management office
Area military and local federal facilities
National Guard
U.S. Department of Energy
Federal Bureau of Investigation
Public Health Service
Centers for Disease Control and Prevention
Environmental Protection Agency
U.S. Coast Guard
Representatives of neighboring jurisdictions

The list is not intended to be either prescriptive or inclusive.

Instructor's Background Information on the Incident

This scenario involving terrorism with a chemical weapon of mass destruction (WMD) portrays an incident that local response groups and agencies can use to evaluate their coordination and response capabilities. They may also identify shortfalls in personnel or other resources that can be supplemented by state or federal sources. The scenario is intended to portray only the hypothetical technical features of a chemical terrorism incident and does not represent an actual event.

This scenario takes place in [*city, state*]. [*A brief description of the location of the chemical incident, a shopping mall located within the jurisdiction participating in this activity. If the mall is named, use the proper name and highlight some of the major tenants. The mall selected, if more than one is available, should be the one closest to the center of town or major traffic arteries. The description should also include information on the number of shoppers found at the mall on an average day.*]

In this scenario, a terrorist group has obtained 8 gallons of the nerve agent sarin (GB is the international military symbol)) and puts this liquid nerve agent into four 2-gallon pressurized metal containers with aerosol release valves. The mall ventilation system carries the agent throughout the mall and to surrounding parking lots, where it will not survive for very long. The release has the potential to affect everyone within the mall and a large number of people in the surrounding area.

The effects of a sarin release of this form (aerosol) are instantaneous. These include blurred vision, breathing difficulty, gastrointestinal distress, skeletal muscle paralysis, seizures, loss of consciousness, and death.

The four sarin containers are placed inside open-top trash cans inside the mall. These are simultaneously released during the height of the lunch hour, when the mall experiences its peak occupancy for the day. The terrorists placed the canisters in the outer-perimeter hallways of the first floor of the mall, effectively blocking ground-level entrances. The release disperses the sarin from each canister into the atmosphere, directly contaminating many people.

In this scenario, it should be apparent that a nerve agent is involved. However, responders cannot identify the type of agent released. Thus, for the purposes of this scenario, consider decontamination aspects. The medics responding to the scene have Occupational Safety and Health Administration training and should recognize some of the symptoms. If not, the sequence of events and the massive number of casualties should indicate that a gas release has occurred.

Vehicular access to the incident site (the mall) is complicated by the fact that the release spawns general panic, leading to spontaneous evacuation of the surrounding area. Responders should know their limitations. Moreover, unaware of the presence of gas upon arrival, many of the first responders are exposed to the sarin.

At some point, it should be obvious that the casualties require decontamination before they can be treated by unprotected medical personnel or before casualties can be allowed to depart the area. Furthermore, casual exposure to the nerve agent increases the number of casualties. In the case of sarin (a nonpersistent agent) this is **NOT** a major issue; however, it must be seriously considered. Persons exposed to very small amounts of the nerve agent show limited symptoms and can be successfully treated if the symptoms are noted in time and the proper antidotes (especially atropine) are available. One should expect, however, countless individuals exhibiting symptoms based on stress and hysteria rather than actual exposure.

It should be easy to determine that this is a terrorism incident. As such, the Federal Bureau of Investigation (FBI) must be notified. The instructor should explore how this notification will take place. This also raises many command and control issues that will be explored further in Session II.

The evaluator should customize Scene I on the following pages and provide it to each of the participants.

Scene I: The WMD Event Occurs

[*City, state, of the incident in the scenario*], [*day of week, date of the incident in the scenario*]. The weather forecast predicts [*insert the weather forecast for the scenario within the normal range for the date of the exercise; include the daily temperature range, the amount of cloud cover, and the wind speed and direction; if possible, set up the scenario for a calm, cool, overcast day*]. At midday it is [*temperature, in degrees Fahrenheit, within the forecasted range*].

At 12:15 p.m. (1215 hours), the [*name of the mall involved in the incident in the scenario*] is filled with lunch-hour shoppers, and the surrounding parking areas are congested with higher than normal levels of traffic.

At 12:30 p.m. (1230 hours), a 911 dispatcher receives a call from the [*name of mall*] security manager ([*name of security manager*]). He or she reports that hundreds of customers inside the mall are gasping for air and convulsing. Hundreds more are collapsing. He or she is evacuating the mall and needs help. First responders are immediately dispatched to the scene. Within minutes, other callers report seeing people collapsed outside the [*name of the mall*].

After dispatching emergency units to the site, the 911 center notifies the municipal switchboard. Reports of casualties at the mall follow. Fire and police squads and medical emergency units arrive on site and initiate emergency response operations. The [*title and name of the chief executive of the jurisdiction, e.g., Mayor John Smith of Central City*] is notified that a crisis of potentially major proportions is unfolding. Major highways and access roads are congested with heavier than normal traffic and scattered traffic collisions in the immediate area caused by individuals fleeing the mall after seeing people collapse, making the response more difficult.

People inside the mall and in the parking lots near the building exits and vents appear to have been exposed to an unidentified substance and are convulsing and asphyxiating. Some are shaking uncontrollably and sweating profusely. Many appear dead, and others who are severely incapacitated require immediate medical assistance. Victims are transported to area hospitals, but some first responders at the response site exhibit similar symptoms and need immediate medical attention. Residential areas in the surrounding areas appear to be unaffected.

At 1:45 p.m. (1345 hours) the state Emergency Operations Center (EOC) in [*location of state EOC*] is activated. At 2:15 p.m. (1415 hours), a representative from the news division of [*name of local television station*] contacts city officials to report that an unidentified caller claims to have released a nerve agent at [*name of the mall*] that afternoon as the first part of a coordinated terrorist attack against [*incident city*]. The television station goes live with the story moments later.

By 3:30 p.m. (1530 hours), the emergency departments at [*names of all medical centers, hospitals, or major trauma facilities*] report that some of their personnel exhibit the same symptoms as patients from the mall. [*The name of the second largest medical center or hospital in the area*] reports that its emergency department is operating at full capacity, that it has activated its mass-casualty disaster plan, and that it is unable to care for additional victims. Designated trauma centers request technical information regarding the agent used in the terrorist attack. Medical collection points are established around [*at least two named locations located a minimum of two blocks upwind from the mall*]. [*The name of the largest medical center or hospital in the area*] reports that tissue and blood samples from several of the victims were packaged as extreme biohazards. The samples were sent to the [*appropriate advanced forensics, academic, or hazardous materials (hazmat) laboratory in the area or region; it should be reachable within a couple of hours, if possible*] by special courier.

National television broadcasts linking with local affiliates show live pictures of the incapacitated and the dead being removed from the mall. Reporters request information regarding the city's response to and preparedness for this type of incident. A major national cable news network requests an interview with a representative from the city.

Residents within 2 miles of the affected mall spontaneously evacuate their homes, frightened by the images on television. Traffic bottlenecks form on all major city transportation arteries, including [*name of one or two major transportation arteries normally used during emergency responses*], further complicating response activities. The combination of spontaneous evacuees and above-normal levels of traffic result in virtual gridlock throughout the area.

Facilitated Discussion

Purpose

This guided group discussion is designed to help participants understand the types of issues that they will encounter and the conflicts across agencies and jurisdictions that can occur in coordinating, communicating, and responding to such an incident. It also gives participants an opportunity to assess their jurisdiction's ability to respond to such an incident.

Presentation

Provide participants with a copy of the questions that does not include the answers to questions, additional questions, or the final note to the facilitator.

Guide a group discussion by asking the numbered questions on the following pages. These questions are not all inclusive; use them to develop additional questions, as necessary. Some additional questions are included should there be a need to stimulate further discussion.

Don't forget that good facilitators speak much less than the participants. This is an assessment activity, not a formal instructional class.

Be sure to touch on the following areas: direction and control, notification and activation, communications, warning and emergency public information, hazard assessment, and management of field response.

Questions, Scene I

1. How will you learn of this incident involving a WMD? What internal and external notifications should you make? Are you satisfied that the current notification process is timely and adequate?

Each jurisdiction and agency should have notification procedures outlined in their emergency operations plans (EOPs). The EOP review completed by the facilitator during the development portion of this activity should provide adequate detail to support facilitated discussion. The following provides general guidance:

–In many jurisdictions, the 911 dispatcher serves as the hub of the notification system and notifies agencies and/or individuals.

–In most jurisdictions, the police and fire departments have excellent internal notification systems; however, other participating agencies may not. Check this during the EOP review. During the discussion explore if or how the police and fire departments could assist other agencies.

–Walk participants through each step of the notification and activation process. Let them estimate their time of arrival and where they will be reporting. Do they anticipate any traffic, transportation, or communication delays that could significantly affect their response? Is there a system in place to facilitate notification when individuals are out of the office, for example, at lunch or at a meeting? How would the lower levels of staffing normally associated with the lunch hour affect the notification process?

Follow-up Questions:

Does your jurisdiction have a policy that prevents full activation of the emergency management system when it is not needed?

The screening process should be defined in local EOPs and often relies on the local office of emergency management or the EOC (if it is staffed 24 hours a day) to serve as the decision maker.

Who handles notification of state and federal authorities?

The responsibility for notification of the state and federal authorities should be clearly defined in the local plan. For an incident of this magnitude, the National Response Center should be notified.

If this incident involving a WMD actually occurred, how long would it take responders to arrive on the scene? How long would it be before an incident command (or other management) structure is established?

Each agency present should provide estimates, and the participants should try to reach a consensus on the overall response time.

Explore with the participants when or what staffing level constitutes a management structure that is operational.

2. How will identification of the presence of hazardous materials occur? How will confirmation of the type of chemical hazard occur?

The EOP review should provide details on how the hazardous materials team (HMT) identifies "unknown agents," because it is unlikely that the local team could readily identify sarin. Supporting laboratories in the area should have been preidentified and agreed to support jurisdictional emergency response operations. Additional information can be obtained by the following:

–M-1 Chemical Agent Detector Paper and the M256 Chemical Agent Detector Kit can both identify the presence of nerve agents. Both are commonly used by military units; however, most fire departments and hazmat units are not equipped with this technology and must be cautious when using it. Query the group to see if they know how to obtain the materials. The M256 kit is more effective for identifying sarin because it is designed to primarily detect vapor hazards.

–The HMT should carry mine safety association detector tubes or similar systems that will capture a sample of the air; however, these will NOT make a positive identification of the presence of a nerve agent.

Follow-up Questions:

Will responders and/or hazmat units recognize the symptoms associated with nerve agents? Will responders test the air before responding?

The answers to these questions should be indicated through review of the EOP and the discussion associated with Question 3 below. Here, issues such as response, protection of the population, and rescue versus self-preservation and maintenance of a response capability should be addressed (i.e., responders should not be used as detectors or allowed to become victims).

3. What information, equipment, and actions are required by your jurisdiction to conduct the initial assessment of the incident? How do you anticipate that information will be distributed among responders?

Include the following items in your discussion:

–a method to determine the identity of the agent,
–a method to determine the extent or area of contamination, and
–a method to determine the decontamination requirements.

4. What immediate decisions related to protective actions that should be taken should the jurisdiction make? How will they be implemented?

Decision making related to the protective actions that should be taken is a critical issue, and the participants should be allowed sufficient time to discuss the ramifications of their decisions. The whole issue of evacuation versus sheltering should be explored. The EOP should provide a framework for making such decisions. In the case of sarin because it poses a significant vapor hazard, sheltering is not an appropriate response. The immediate area, adjacent buildings, and the hazardous area downwind should be evacuated.

Allow participants to discuss the issues of decontamination and triage strategies.

Follow-up Questions:

Should the surrounding area be evacuated in this case, or will sheltering be an appropriate response?

Should the jurisdiction be concerned about the possibility of additional attacks?

This is always a possibility, and the participants in the group should discuss what changes they will have to make to manage additional incidents of either a terrorism event involving a WMD or more common emergencies (e.g., fires and auto collisions).

What medical facilities are victims and patients being sent to?

What types of information should the emergency medical service units relay to the hospitals in the area to prepare them to receive potentially contaminated patients? Should any areas be quarantined?

These questions focus on the initial medical response. Allow the participants to discuss this topic, if they bring it up. If discussion of this topic is not initiated by the participants, it will be fully examined during the discussion associated with Scene II.

5. How will the incident site be secured to ensure that the crime scene is protected and no contaminated personnel or equipment leave the area? What access and egress control procedures should be implemented?

The EOP should provide details on contamination control procedures and crime scene protection as part of its WMD annex, if it exists. The EOP review should also provide an indication of how the jurisdiction will manage these issues.

Allow the participants in the group to discuss their security procedures and how these relate to their overall response strategy.

Access and egress control procedures should be included in the hazmat portion of the local plan. Determine the group's understanding of the importance of this issue.

6. Is the current number of trained, qualified personnel within your jurisdiction sufficient to respond to this incident? If not, where will you seek support to bridge these deficiencies?

A review of the EOP should provide an indication of the number of trained and qualified personnel.

Mutual-support agreements with other local governments and state agencies should be discussed at this point.

The National Strike Force and the Army Technical Escort Unit are among the federal agencies with expertise in this area.

7. Will the city or county EOC be adequate for coordination of the response to this incident? Will a separate command center that is physically close to the incident site be required? What resources are available for outfitting this command center?

This information should be extracted from the EOP. It is assumed that an incident command system will be used.

Follow-up Questions:

How long will it take to have an EOC activated and fully operational? What are the capabilities of the center? Are these capabilities adequate to respond to an incident of the magnitude presented here?

In this scenario, the command post should be at the local EOC, so the answer will depend on how long it will take to activate the EOC and staff it appropriately and on whether the local EOC is in the affected area. If so, the use of an alternate site should be discussed.

The capabilities of the local EOC and an alternate EOC should be apparent from the plan review.

Note that these are not all-encompassing questions. They are only a starting point. Other issues that the jurisdiction must be capable of dealing with may arise. If topics that are more closely associated with the following two scenes are brought up, table that discussion until the appropriate time.

Instructor's Background Information on the Incident, Scene II

The FBI attempts to establish control of the situation for crisis management, that is, a criminal investigation. At the same time, the scope of the situation makes it clear that there is also a federal role for consequence management. The Federal Emergency Management Agency (FEMA) is the federal agency designated to manage the consequence management aspect of the incident. The participants are probably not well versed in the difference between the federal definitions of crisis management and consequence management.

The presence of a nerve agent is established. Sarin is the prime suspect, although it is not confirmed by laboratory analysis. The nonpersistence of sarin means that much of the response effort takes place during the first 6 hours. Sarin dissipates after 3 or 4 hours in open areas, but it may linger in confined spaces, creating hot spots. Because the identification of the agent is unconfirmed, responders should follow response strategies associated with persistent agents.

The highways experience tremendous gridlock, and hospitals run out of medications; generally, a state of chaos persists. Consider the difficulties associated with decontaminating all of the individuals involved in the deliberate and spontaneous evacuations and those involved with the response and the consequences of failing to do so.

The large number of casualties (400 dead and 2,00 other people with severe symptoms) in this scenario quickly exhausts the limited supply of medicines such as atropine. The triage referenced in the scenario is a practice in which the emphasis is on saving the lives of as many people as possible, which means that individuals who are likely to die or for whom heroic efforts will be required to save them are lower in the treatment priority than individuals who can be more expeditiously treated.

During this session participants should recognize that federal assistance, whether it is wanted or not, is on the way. The local and state response capabilities are overwhelmed. The challenge is integrating the local response with federal and state interests and capabilities. The criminal investigation, coordinated by the FBI, has the potential to conflict with the humanitarian aspects of the response.

A host of federal agencies are potentially involved. They include the Environmental Protection Agency, the U.S. Department of Health and Human Services, the U.S. Department of Transportation, and most importantly, the U.S. Department of Defense because the Army has the greatest expertise in dealing with treatment and decontamination of individuals who have come into contact with chemical agents. In an actual situation it can be a real challenge to sort out all the different agencies involved in the response. A very important nonfederal agency is the American Red Cross, which offers invaluable assistance in dealing with family notification and reunification issues, as well as shelter operation.

The resources most likely required from the state National Guard are transportation, communications, and security, as well as expertise and resources related to chemical warfare.

Scene II: Chaos in the City

It is still [*day of week, date of the incident in the scenario*] in [*city, state, of the incident in the scenario*]. The weather remains calm and cloudy. The temperature is currently [*high temperature, in degrees Fahrenheit, forecast for the scenario*].

At 4:30 p.m. (1630 hours), the [*name of the local airport*] is shut down by the airport's director of aviation following the imposition of a widespread "no-fly" area over the city by the Federal Aviation Administration. The airport will remain closed until further notice.

A preliminary situation report indicates that 400 people are dead and the unidentified hazmat has affected 2,000 other people at the [*name of the mall*] and surrounding area. Residents in the vicinity request directions to shelters as they evacuate. There is mounting concern and fear over the potential for additional chemical agent releases in other areas of the city. Media reports include rumors of widespread panic.

Responders continue to assess protective measures. Hot spots are identified inside the mall's ventilation system and other confined spaces. Responders evaluate containment and decontamination strategies at these hot spots and ask if "forced ventilation" is an option. Evacuation of selected areas continues. Other measures that can be used to protect the public are evaluated. Hazmat responders debate declaring up-wind areas around the release sites safe for reentry and believe that vapor or inhalation risk is a threat in a limited area. Designated shelter locations request food, medicine, and dwelling resources and information on containment actions to prevent the spread of contamination with the chemical agent to clean areas.

Hospitals in the area report increasing cases of medical personnel exhibiting symptoms of exposure. Medical teams are unsuccessful in identifying a chemical nerve agent, although they are certain that symptoms are caused by organophosphate poisoning. Because of the symptoms manifested by its medical personnel, [*the name of the second largest medical center or hospital in the area*] closes its emergency department and discourages people from coming to its facility. The [*name of the second largest medical center or hospital in the area*] director calls the city requesting assistance in evacuating unexposed hospital patients to another medical facility.

Area morgues are overwhelmed. Requests are made for additional resources to manage the number of bodies removed from the incident locations. The [*city, county*] EOC requests chemical decontamination assistance from the state and FEMA. Concerned relatives, desperate for information regarding the fate of their loved ones, call the local hospitals and cause the local telephone exchange to overload and fail.

At 5 p.m. (1700 hours), Governor [*last name of the state governor*] declares a state of emergency and formally requests a presidential declaration of a major disaster. Pending the president's decision on whether to declare a disaster, the governor asks for implementation of Section 403(C) of the Stafford Act. The White House is briefed on the incident. Federal officials are notified, and federal agency regional representatives are directed to [*city of the incident in the scenario; if the federal regional headquarters is within a 1-hour drive of the incident site, federal representatives may already be on site*].

The [*appropriate advanced forensics, academic, or hazmat laboratory in the area or region*] calls the [*name of state*] emergency management agency (EMA) and the city to indicate that it has identified the chemical agent as sarin, the same substance used by Japanese cult members in their attack on the Tokyo subway in 1995.

A FEMA Region [*region number*] representative (or the federal coordinating officer) requests that the [*name of state*] EMA identify potential locations for the Disaster Field Office. The Disaster Field Office coordinates the overall response in accordance with the Federal Response Plan. The [*name of state*] EMA coordinates with the [*city or county*] EOC to determine the best sites for establishment of the Disaster Field Office. An advanced emergency response team is on its way from FEMA headquarters in Washington, D.C.

At 7 p.m. (1900 hours), a U.S. Department of Transportation spokesperson announces that the incident in [*city, state, of incident scenario*] is disrupting the national transportation network. [*Provide a list of possible impacts on the national transportation network, e.g.:*

if the mall is near Amtrak or other rail transportation lines, it could halt rail transportation along a major corridor;

if the local airport is a major transportation hub or if its closure could affect a major transportation hub, its closure could cause major disruptions of air traffic; and

the gridlock status of the Interstate highways through the area could cause disruption to Interstate traffic along major trucking corridors.]

An FBI terrorist team is dispatched to [*city of the incident in the scenario*] to direct crisis management operations. The team director is scheduled to meet with the [*city or county*] EOC and [*name of state*] EMA directors upon arrival. The area FBI representative arrives on site and takes control of the investigation. FBI officials suspect a terrorist group may be responsible for the incident in [*city, state, of the incident in the scenario*].

At 8 p.m. (2000 hours), media groups interview emergency response experts. Some theorize that the level of sophistication in the attack is an indication of international assistance. The group points to similarities between this incident and that on the Tokyo subway.

Questions, Scene II

1. Who is in charge of the incident site? How will your agency's actions be coordinated with the actions of other agencies? What conflicts could arise from the need to simultaneously conduct extensive criminal investigatory and response functions? What conflicts may be anticipated between the overlapping federal, state, and local jurisdictions?

Explore the federal definitions of crisis management and consequence management. At the federal level, the FBI has authority over the incident site and is responsible for crisis management. FEMA has federal authority for consequence management but must conform to the direction of the FBI to protect as much of the crime scene as possible while assisting state and local authorities with providing the needed rescue and relief to protect the population. It is anticipated that most jurisdictions will follow this delineation of responsibilities.

Determine who is in charge of the local response for both consequence and crisis management.

Determine the command or management structure to be used by the jurisdiction. The incident command system has been adapted by many jurisdictions as their command structure during response operations. Explore the specifics of the local system during this discussion. A review of the EOP should have provided details on the structure of the command structure.

Conflicts will likely be related to the jurisdiction's attempt to balance protecting evidence and protecting people. Overlapping conflicts can occur as state and federal responders arrive on scene and the transition to a unified, joint, or coordinated command or management structure begins.

2. What community health planning has been completed? Have privately owned hospitals, home-care agencies, long-term-care facilities, and clinics been incorporated into the EOP and included in the planning process? Has your community conducted joint exercises for this type or any type of mass-casualty situation?

The EOP review should indicate the preparedness of the community health program to address mass-casualty situations and the involvement of all local health care assets in the planning process.

Most jurisdictions should have been involved in joint mass-casualty exercises because these are an accreditation requirement for most health care organizations, especially hospitals.

Follow-up Questions:

What on-scene medical operations might be necessary?

This issue should be addressed in the community health plan as it exists. The priorities at the scene should be gross triage, transportation, and limited lifesaving efforts.

Will triage stations be established? Where will these be established?

The discussion of triage should focus on managing the flow of casualties through the community health system. The community health plan should address this issue.

What types of communications should be conducted between responders and the hospitals before the arrival of exposed victims? How will exposed patients be processed at the point of collection and the point of delivery?

Communications protocols for providing critical information should be provided within the communications section of the EOP.

Triage protocols at both collection and delivery points should also be part of the plan. Basic requirements dictate that triage be performed at both locations. This may be a good point to address the differences between standard emergency department triage and mass-casualty triage.

What medical resource shortfalls do you anticipate? What specific assistance do you need from the state and federal governments? How will these resources be integrated into the response operations?

Adequate amounts of nerve agent antidotes and sufficient numbers of medical personnel resources are the most obvious shortfalls.

State and federal plans provide for mobilization of these types of resources in disaster situations. It is important for the participants to realize that there may be a significant time delay before those resources are available.

What type of epidemiological surveillance program does your community have in place? How well defined are the linkages between the

community health program and plan and your consequence management infrastructure?

Epidemiological surveillance is important in determining the number of individuals who were exposed to the nerve agent. Community health planning should account for locating within the incident area personnel who may be asymptomatic at this point.

The EOP should define the linkage between the community health program and the emergency operations management structure, and a representative of the community health agency or emergency medical service should be on the management team.

3. What immediate public relations and media concerns must be anticipated? How will these concerns be addressed? Who will serve as your jurisdiction's spokesperson in this incident?

The Joint Information Center should be established after the arrival of state and federal assets and should serve as the source of pubic information after that point. The plan should identify who will serve as the local spokesperson before the establishment of the Joint Information Center.

Most EOPs assign the management of public affairs issues to the management team located in the EOC. Determine participants' familiarity with public affairs procedures. Anticipating that public panic and extreme fear are likely to exist, the group should discuss how to diffuse the issue without denigrating the seriousness of the situation. Determine if the participants understand the importance of a multimedia approach and the development of themes.

In the early stages of a response, public safety messages must be disseminated quickly.

Follow-up Question:

Does the communications system meet the multilingual needs of the area?

The EOP review should identify the multilingual needs of the community and procedures for meeting those needs

4. What are the internal and external communications requirements for this response? Who is responsible for ensuring that the necessary systems are available? What problems may be anticipated?

The EOP should address internal and external communications requirements and assign responsibility for maintaining a viable system. Communications support equipment is normally located in or adjacent to the EOC.

Internal communications issues focus on the ability of jurisdictions to communicate with responders from different agencies (e.g., fire departments talking to police). Determine what system is in place to facilitate such coordination or if coordination must be accomplished face to face, through dispatchers, or through the EOC.

External communications issues should focus on the procedures for providing essential information to state and federal responders and managers who are en route to the incident site.

Solutions that rely on public hard telephone lines or cellular telephone systems should be discouraged in light of the numerous demands that will be made on those systems, unless the plan review revealed that a priority override system for emergency communications is in place with local telephone service providers.

Instructor's Background Information on the Incident, Scene III

It is now 9 hours after the initial releases. At this point, the FBI has effectively established control of the situation for crisis management purposes. The casualty figures are horrendous: 400 dead and 2,000 more people with severe symptoms. The only good news is that it is unlikely there will be many additional casualties, as it has been determined that the agent released was nonpersistent sarin. However, the threat of additional releases still looms until the terrorist group makes a formal statement to the contrary. At this point, adequate amounts of atropine have been rushed to the scene and to treatment centers.

The response has required all of the city's emergency response forces and most of those available from the neighboring counties and other nearby cities. The stress and trauma of dealing with death on such a large scale are affecting many of the responders at the scene. Crew relief schedules have not been worked out at this time.

Decontamination is expected not to be a major issue anymore, except to foster public confidence. Cleanup and restoration of services will and should last at least 1 week.

Scene III: The Immediate Threat Wanes

It is still [*day, date of the incident in the scenario*] in [*city, state, of the incident in the scenario*]. The sun went down at [*appropriate time*]. The weather remains calm and cloudy. The temperature is currently [*forecasted evening temperature, in degrees Fahrenheit*].

The number of bodies collected overwhelms the city and surrounding morgues. Shelters are activated and provide emergency services to evacuees and displaced people. Hospitals report a noticeable drop in the number of additional victims arriving at these facilities; however, hysterical patients and asymptomatic victims continue to arrive. Mutual aid from across the country continues, increasing the need for coordination of resource allocation. National FEMA and FBI representatives are on scene.

Concerned residents overload the phone emergency switchboard with requests for information regarding the whereabouts of family members. Media representatives transmit live interviews from [*city of the incident*]. Residents are reluctant to return to their homes, despite assurances that designated areas are safe for reentry. National attention is focused on [*city of the incident*]. The incident sends shock waves through the country. People nationwide avoid public places.

At 10 p.m. (2200 hours), the president issues a major disaster declaration granting FEMA authority to provide emergency response support to [*city of the incident*] and to conduct consequence management activities. The president, in a special statement to the nation carried live on all networks, condemns the vile act of terrorism and vows to punish the culprits. The Disaster Field Office, with its additional federal resources, will not be fully operational for another 24 hours.

It is anticipated that the [*complete name of the mall where the incident occurred*] and the immediate vicinity will remain closed until it is declared safe for public use (at least 1 week). The FBI directs that general, deliberate bomb searches be conducted for all major public gathering places. Although there have been no further calls from the terrorist organization, the FBI takes the statement that characterized the attack "as the first part of a coordinated terrorist attack against [*the city of the incident*]" during the 2:15 p.m. (1415 hours) call to [*local television station listed in Scene I*] very seriously.

The [*name of the local airport*] will reopen in the morning, but many scheduled flights into the area during the next few days are cancelled. Local businesspeople raise the specter of an economic slowdown because of concerns that their inability to resume normal operations will have a negative impact on their business activity, especially in light of the generalized searches being conducted.

Planning for site decontamination, remediation, and cleanup is initiated. Coordination of response efforts over the next 48 hours continues. Questions related to medical surveillance of response team members and the population at large, the decision to authorize population reentry, as well as public security issues, long-term medical support services, and implementation of recovery plans, are open for discussion.

Questions, Scene III

1. How will you conduct extended response operations? Are local personnel and equipment resources adequate for the extended operations that will be required?

The EOP should account for around-the-clock operations. Many jurisdictions plan to send a portion of the EOC staff home after the initial incident assessment reveals the need for extended operations. Determine who will be responsible for each function on multiple shifts.

Each agency will likely be overwhelmed. The real question is how much state, federal, National Guard, and mutual-aid support is needed.

2. What are your procedures for integrating state and federal resources into your management organization?

The EOP should outline the procedures for integration of state and federal resources.

State and federal assistance is supplementary to the local response; and as the Disaster Field Office is established, the federal coordinating officer and the state coordinating officer (SCO) will coordinate the activities of the state and local governments, the American Red Cross, the Salvation Army, and other disaster relief organizations.

Follow-up Questions:

How will your agency coordinate its action with other agencies (federal, state, and local) and public interest groups?

The federal coordinating officer is the primary federal coordinating authority for consequence management; the FBI handles crisis management.

With the arrival of state and federal assistance and the formation of a Joint Information Center, how will media inquiries be handled? Who in your jurisdiction is responsible for authoring media releases?

Media releases must be coordinated with the FBI, FEMA, and state and local authorities once the Joint Information Center has been established.

The EOP should provide a detailed communications and public relations plan.

3. What continuing assessments should be enacted when the cleanup phase is complete? Who will make these determinations?

Long-range health issues should be of some concern, although in the case of sarin, these will most likely be psychosomatic health issues.

4. What are the environmental concerns related to this incident?

No environmental concerns should be expected from the sarin itself; however, the local responders might identify some issues particular to their area of work.

Materials encountered or used during the response will continue to present hazards until they are neutralized.

Follow-up Questions:

What steps will be taken by your agency to ensure adequate sanitation measures throughout the affected area?

The local hazmat plan should identify sanitation procedures.

What local requirements exist for reentry to an area evacuated because of a hazmat incident?

The hazmat annex to the EOP should outline procedures for reentry into an evacuated area.

After the use of chemical agents, the local emergency management team should consider the need for "safe certification," that is, having a third-party laboratory verify that the area is free from contamination.

5. Within your jurisdiction, what psychological traumas may be anticipated? How will your agency deal with these traumas?

Many agencies have teams already designated to assist in such cases. In most instances, the teams will not have the capacity to handle the expected number of cases in an incident of this magnitude.

Discuss the availability of crisis counseling. Also, refer participants to Section 416 of the Stafford Act.

Follow-up Questions:

How will your agency participate in notification of the deaths of civilians and your colleagues? Are personnel in your agency adequately trained in the process of death notification?

Death notification is always a difficult issue. The EOP should provide guidance to managers. However, at a minimum someone in the supervisory chain should be involved with the actual notification.

RADIOLOGICAL SCENARIO (PLUTONIUM)

Potential Participants

Fire department
Police department or sheriff's office
Office of Emergency Services
Public works department
Public health department
Public information officer
General counsel's office
Medical examiner or coroner's office
Emergency department physician
Transportation authority (port authority, airport authority, etc.)
Coordinator of volunteer organizations
Emergency medical service
Hazardous materials team
State emergency management office
Area military and local federal facilities
National Guard
U.S. Department of Energy
Federal Bureau of Investigation
Public Health Service
Centers for Disease Control and Prevention
Environmental Protection Agency
U.S. Coast Guard
Representatives of neighboring jurisdictions

The list is not intended to be either prescriptive or inclusive.

Instructor's Background Information on the Incident, Scene I

This radiological terrorism scenario portrays an incident that local response groups and agencies can use to evaluate their coordination and response capabilities. They may also identify shortfalls in personnel or other resources that can be supplemented by state or federal sources. The scenario is intended to portray only the hypothetical technical features of a radiological terrorism incident and does not represent an actual event.

This scenario takes place in [*city, state*]. [*Provide a brief description of the location of the radiological incident. If the building is named, then use the proper name and highlight some of the major tenants in the building.*] [*The location for this event should be near the middle of town in a multistory building that houses some type of hazardous materials (hazmats). A building with a propane tank on its roof or stores of compressed gases is especially attractive because either will support an initiation of the radiological terrorism incident. If possible, locate the incident so that it will affect multiple transportation nodes by selecting a building that is in close proximity to a navigable river, an Interstate highway, a subway system, and an airport. Location of the incident in a building with federal or state government offices or in the area of the offices of any law enforcement authority is another desirable characteristic.*]

[*Provide a brief description of any local hazards that might complicate the response to the incident and its initial accompanying fires.*]

[*The incident should occur during a period with high levels of traffic at or on the proximate traffic nodes. Provide a description of the normal traffic patterns in the area.*]

Highlights of this scene include the following:

Terrorists detonate a tank of compressed flammable gas with a device around which 600 grams of plutonium-238 is wrapped, with the radioactivity dispersed at the time of the explosion.

Responders to the scene are unaware of the presence of radioactive material for approximately 1 hour and 40 minutes.

Hazmat teams, while normally equipped with CDV-750/1500 radioactivity survey meters, may not use them unless they know of a radioactive threat.

Because of the proximity of large quantities of hazmats to the explosion, many responders are called in.

The terrorist group responsible for the detonation calls [*call sign of a local news radio station*] to report the explosion and radioactive release.

The local news radio station reports the explosion and the possibility of a radioactive release, causing widespread panic.

Spontaneous evacuation creates traffic chaos and overwhelms police.

The state and the National Response Center are notified of the incident.

Responders are challenged to

- Determine what type of radioactive material was used in the attack.
- Initiate appropriate decontamination procedures for the victims.
- Provide appropriate protection to responders on scene.
- Prevent the spread of the material from contaminated persons who spontaneously evacuated from the affected area.
- Arrange for fast medical treatment for victims.

For people in the general population, national guidelines recommend dose limits of 0.5 rem/year, although international guidelines set dose limits of 0.5 rem/year for short-term exposure and 0.1 rem/year for long-term exposure. Gamma radiation travels the farthest and can penetrate the entire body. It takes about 90 years for one-half of a quantity of plutonium-238 to break down to its daughter chemicals and about 24,000 years for plutonium-239 to do the same.

It should be easy to determine that this is a terrorism incident. As such, the Federal Bureau of Investigation (FBI) must be notified.

The instructor should explore how this notification will take place. This also raises many command and control issues that will be explored in further detail during Sessions II and III.

Scene I: The WMD Event Occurs

[*City, state, of the incident in the scenario*], [*day of week, date of the incident in the scenario*]. The weather forecast predicts [*insert the weather forecast for the scenario; make the temperature range, amount of cloud cover, wind speed, and wind direction within the normal ranges for the date of the exercise. Wind speed and direction should be manipulated to allow the radioactive fallout to cause the desired impact on the city. Include a threat of evening rain in the forecast.*]. At [*time of the incident; an artificial time, not the start time of the exercise, but one selected to provide greater impact on the exposed population*] it is [*temperature, in degrees Fahrenheit, within the forecasted range*].

At 12:35 p.m. (1235 hours), a series of loud explosions is heard at the [*building or area of the incident*]. A minute later, 911 receives a call from [*the building tenants*] and is informed that two 1,000-gallon aboveground propane storage tanks and a 3,000-gallon aboveground liquid oxygen tank (within 100 feet of the propane tanks) have exploded. Several buildings and two vehicles ignited as a result of debris from the explosions and are burning. At least one building in the area has major structural damage and is on the verge of collapse. The caller mentions that he and 4 other employees were able to evacuate the site but that 10 employees are dead and 6 are not accounted for. The caller gives the operator the address of the incident site.

The fire and police departments are called to the scene of the fire. Within minutes, firefighters, police officers, and other emergency rescue teams arrive on the scene. The fire threatens [*provide a description of nearby facilities, especially hazmat sites, e.g., a nearby oil tank farm, power plant, or government office building*].

Upon arrival at the scene, police evacuate the area and close the road. The initial incident commander calls in a second and third alarm due to the magnitude of the fire and the additional hazmat threat. A large black cloud develops over the area of the fire, swelling in size as the wind moves it [*direction of cloud drift based on wind direction; provide direction to, not direc-*

tion from, as wind direction is normally reported] of the incident site. By this time, emergency management team notifications are initiated and the [*jurisdiction*]'s Emergency Operations Center (EOC) is activated.

At 1:15 p.m. (1315 hours), a dispatcher with the police department receives a call from a news producer at [*call sign of a local news radio station*]. The station received a call at approximately 1 p.m. (1300 hours) from an unidentified individual claiming responsibility for setting off a nuclear device at [*address of incident location and building name*].

At 1:30 p.m. (1330 hours), [*call sign of a local news radio station*] airs a report about the explosion and announces that a terrorist group claims responsibility for planting a nuclear device at the explosion site. The newscaster notes that the police and FBI have not confirmed their report and will provide information as it becomes available. As news of the explosion and the possibility of a radioactive material release become more widely known, people around the site of the fire and in and around the downtown area panic and flee. This spontaneous evacuation causes traffic gridlock throughout the downtown area and along [*Interstate and other highway designators, e.g., I-XX and Highway X*].

By 2 p.m. (1400 hours), both the [*city name*] and the state EOC are activated. The National Response Center is notified of the explosions and the possibility of a radioactive release.

Facilitated Discussion

Purpose

This guided group discussion is designed to help participants understand the types of issues that they will encounter and the conflicts across agencies and jurisdictions that can occur in coordinating, communicating, and responding to such an incident. It also gives participants an opportunity to assess their jurisdiction's ability to respond to such an incident.

Presentation

Guide a group discussion by asking the numbered questions on the following pages. These questions are not all inclusive; use them to develop additional questions, as necessary. Some additional questions are included should there be a need to stimulate further discussion.

Don't forget that good facilitators speak much less than the participants. This is an assessment activity, not a formal instructional class.

Provide participants with a copy of the questions that does not include the answers to questions, additional questions, or the final note to the facilitator.

Be sure to touch on the following areas: direction and control, notification and activation, communications, warning and emergency public information, hazard assessment, and management of field response.

Questions, Scene I

1. How will you learn of this incident involving a weapon of mass destruction (WMD)? What internal and external notifications should you make? Are you satisfied that the current notification process is timely and adequate?

Each jurisdiction and agency should have notification procedures outlined in their emergency operations plan (EOP). The EOP review completed by the facilitator during the development portion of this activity should provide adequate detail to support facilitated discussion. The following provides general guidance:

- *In many jurisdictions, the 911 dispatcher serves as the hub of the notification system and notifies agencies and individuals.*
- *In most jurisdictions, the police and fire departments have excellent internal notification systems; however, other participating agencies may not. Check this during the EOP review. During the discussion, explore if or how the police and fire departments could assist other agencies.*
- *Walk participants through each step of the notification and activation process. Let them estimate their time of arrival and where they will be reporting. Do they anticipate any traffic, transportation, or communications delays that could significantly affect their response? Is there a system in place to facilitate notification when individuals are out of the office, for example, at lunch or at a meeting? How would the lower staffing normally associated with the lunch hour affect the notification process?*

Follow-up Questions:

Does your jurisdiction have a policy that prevents full activation of the emergency management system when it is not needed?

The screening process should be defined in local EOPs and often relies on the local Office of Emergency Management or the EOC (if it is staffed 24 hours a day) to serve as the decision maker.

Who handles notification of state and federal authorities?

The responsibility for notification of state and federal authorities should be clearly defined in the local plan. For an incident of this magnitude, the National Response Center should be notified.

If this incident involving a WMD occurs, how long will it take responders to arrive on the scene? How long will it be before an incident command (or other management) structure is established?

Each agency present should provide estimates, and the participants should try to reach a consensus on the overall response time.

Explore with the participants when or what staffing level constitutes a management structure that is operational.

2. How will identification of the presence of hazardous materials occur? How will confirmation of the type of chemical hazard occur?

The EOP review should provide details on how the hazmat team identifies unknown agents. Some hazmat teams have received training on identifying radioactive materials and sources of radiation. In this scenario, it is unlikely that the local team would immediately recognize the presence of radioactive material until after the terrorists contacted the radio station. Screening for radioactive material is not part of initial assessment procedures unless there is a strong indication that radioactive materials are present (e.g., a U.S. Department of Transportation hazard placard is present or the material transportation manifest identifies the presence of radioactive materials). Once the team starts looking, it should be able to identify the material as an alpha emitter and may assume that the material is plutonium. Support laboratories in the area should have been preidentified and agreed to support emergency response operations for the jurisdiction. Additional information is provided:

– Some hazmat teams have radiological survey instruments or meters that can detect gamma and beta radiation. All teams may not have alpha radiation detectors; determine the types of instruments on hand within the jurisdiction during the EOP review.

Follow-up Questions:

Will responders and hazmat units recognize the symptoms associated with exposure to radiological materials? Will responders conduct air testing or radiological surveys before responding?

The answers to these questions should be indicated through the EOP review. Here, issues such as response, protection of the population, and rescue versus self-preservation and maintenance of response capability should be addressed (i.e., responders should not be used as detectors or allowed to become victims).

Another topic for discussion at this point is the adequacy of the threat or risk assessment conducted by the local jurisdiction. The management team should be aware of the threats to the community, and their awareness should be based upon a deliberate assessment.

3. What information, equipment, and actions are required by your jurisdiction to conduct the initial assessment of the incident? How do you anticipate information to be distributed among responders?

Include the following items in your discussion:

–a method to determine the size of the radioactivity dispersion device or the amount of plutonium dispersed,

–a method to determine the location and identity of the radioactive material

–survey meters and plume projection models,

–an accurate weather forecast, and

–other methods and actions as reflected in the reference material provided to the participants and developed during the review of the EOP.

4. What immediate decisions related to protective actions that should be taken should the jurisdiction make? How will they be implemented?

Decision making related to the protective actions that should be taken is a critical issue, and the participants should be allowed sufficient time to discuss the ramifications of their decisions. The whole issue of evacuation versus sheltering should be explored. The EOP should provide a framework for making such decisions. In the case of plutonium, sheltering away from the immediate site of the incident is an appropriate response. The immediate area and adjacent buildings should, however, be evacuated due to the risks associated with inhaling particles suspended in the air. Any evacuation must include the use of at least simple respiratory protection.

Allow participants to discuss the issues of decontamination and triage strategies.

Follow-up Questions:

Should the surrounding area be evacuated in this case, or will sheltering be an appropriate response?

Should the jurisdiction be concerned about the possibility of additional attacks?

This is always a possibility, and the group should discuss what changes they will have to make to manage additional incidents of either a terrorist event involving a WMD or more common emergencies (e.g., fires and auto collisions).

What medical facilities are victims and patients being sent to? What types of information should the emergency medical services units relay to the hospitals in the area to prepare them to receive potentially contaminated patients? Should any areas be quarantined?

These questions focus on the initial medical response. Allow the participants to discuss this topic, if they bring it up. If discussion of this topic is not initiated by the participants, it will be fully examined during the discussion associated with Scene II.

5. How will the incident site be secured to ensure that the crime scene is protected and no contaminated personnel or equipment leave the area? What access and egress control procedures should be implemented?

The EOP should provide details on contamination control procedures and crime scene protection as part of its WMD annex, if it exists. The EOP review should also provide an indication of how the jurisdiction will manage these issues.

Allow the participants in the group to discuss their security procedures and how these relate to their overall response strategy.

Access and egress control procedures should be included in the hazmat portion of the local plan. Determine the group's understanding of the importance of this issue.

6. Is the current number of trained, qualified personnel within your jurisdiction sufficient to respond to this incident? If not, where will you seek support to bridge these deficiencies?

A review of the EOP should provide an indication of the number of trained and qualified personnel.

Mutual-support agreements with other local governments and state agencies should be discussed at this point.

The National Strike Force, the U.S. Department of Energy, and the Army Technical Escort Unit are among the federal agencies with expertise in this area.

Another excellent source of assistance to this type of incident is nuclear power plant response teams. (The Radiological Emergency Planning program is an excellent source of information for responding to an incident involving the dispersal of radioactive material.)

7. Will the city or county EOC be adequate for coordinating the response to this incident? Will a separate command center that is physically close to the incident site be required? What resources are available for outfitting this command center?

This information should be extracted from the EOP. It is assumed that an incident command system will be used.

Follow-up Questions:

How long will it take to have an EOC activated and fully operational? What are the capabilities of the center? Are these capabilities adequate to respond to an incident of the magnitude presented here?

In this scenario, the command post should be at the local EOC, so the answer will depend on how long it will take to activate the EOC and staff it appropriately and if the local EOC is in the affected area. If so, the use of an alternate site should be discussed.

The capabilities of the local EOC and alternate EOC should be apparent from the plan review.

Note that these are not all-encompassing questions. They are only a starting point. Other issues that the jurisdiction must be capable of dealing with may arise. If topics that are more closely associated with the following two scenes are brought up, table that discussion until the appropriate time.

Instructor's Background Information on the Incident, Scene II

The FBI attempts to establish control of the situation for crisis management, that is, the criminal investigation. At the same time, the scope of the situation makes it clear there is also a federal role for consequence management. The Federal Emergency Management Agency (FEMA) is the designated federal agency to manage the consequence management aspect of the incident. The participants are probably not well versed in the difference between the federal definitions of crisis management and consequence management.

The presence of radioactive material is established, but indications are that the radioactivity was dispersed via a dispersion device and is not the result of an actual nuclear detonation. Following is information on expected physical reactions to various levels of exposure:

a. 50 rems/hour: redness of the skin

b. 200 rems/hour: blood changes

c. 300 rems/hour: 100 percent of the population experiences nausea, vomiting, and gastrointestinal problems

The therapeutic range of treatment is 100 to 1,000 rems. Rems represent cumulative, whole-body dosage.

FEMA indicates that after 3 hours, people in the fallout area with the highest contamination level suffer radiation sickness and that others will become ill by the 72nd hour. People in the fallout area with lower contamination levels suffer some form of radiation sickness in 3 to 6 hours. In the area of contamination most removed from the explosion, it is unlikely that anyone will suffer radiation sickness within 72 hours.

[*Provide a description of how and where monitoring stations will be set up to monitor people and equipment for contamination based upon the analysis of the EOP. Many jurisdictions may rely on dated "Civil Defense" annexes based on the former Strategic Nuclear Threat.*]

Once it is determined that contamination is an issue, focus the discussion on the next steps. Medical information indicates that removing outer clothing and shoes will, in most cases, effect a 90 to 95 percent reduction in the patient's level of contamination. Patients should be decontaminated as soon as possible, ideally before transfer to a hospital but certainly before admission to a hospital. However, this is not always possible. Therefore, decontamination procedures should be a part of the operational plans and guides of all divisions and departments of medical facilities, not just emergency department or teams.

Because the treatment of injured, contaminated personnel may result in the contamination of almost any part of a medical facility, medical procedures must accomplish the following:

- Minimize the degree of contamination. (*How will they accomplish this?*)
- Identify and measure the extent of the contamination. (*Do they have the equipment and trained personnel?*)
- Remove the contamination. (*How and with which departments will this be coordinated?*)

The removal of contamination is a two-part problem and includes decontamination of people as well as decontamination of equipment and facilities. The former must be started as soon as possible, even if monitoring facilities are not available. Standardized procedures of decontaminating people must be established and instituted. People must not be released before they are monitored and completely decontaminated.

Because plutonium is an alpha particle producer and does not produce a large amount of gamma radiation, harmful health effects are not likely unless the plutonium is breathed or swallowed. Most plutonium exposure occurs through breathing. Once it is breathed in, the amount remaining in the lungs depends on several things, particularly the particle size and form of the plutonium. The forms that dissolve easily may be absorbed (passed through the lungs into other parts of the body), or some may remain in the lungs. The forms that dissolve less easily are often coughed up and then swallowed. However, some of these may also remain in the lungs. The stomach poorly absorbs plutonium taken in with food or water, so most of it leaves the body in feces. Absorption of plutonium through undamaged skin is limited, but it may enter the body through wounds.

During this session participants should recognize that federal assistance, whether it is wanted or not, is on the way. The local response capabilities are overwhelmed. The challenge is integrating the local response with federal and state interests. The criminal investigation, coordinated by the FBI, has the potential to conflict with the humanitarian aspects of the response.

A host of federal agencies are potentially involved. They include the Nuclear Regulatory Commission, the Environmental Protection Agency (EPA), the U.S. Department of Health and Human Services, the U.S. Department of Transportation, and the U.S. Department of Defense. The Nuclear Regulatory Commission and the U.S. Department of Defense are important because they have the greatest expertise with treatment and decontamination of individuals exposed to radioactive materials. Sorting out the agencies involved is a real challenge in an actual situation. An important nonfederal agency is the American Red Cross, which offers assistance in dealing with family notification and reunification issues, as well as assisting stranded travelers.

The resources most likely required from the state are National Guard resources for transportation and security. The National Guard should provide additional monitoring and decontamination equipment resources and operators.

Highlights of this scene include the following:

The presence of radioactive material is confirmed.

Initial readings indicate an exposure level of 60 rems/hour.

Immediate evacuation is ordered.

The FBI informs the EOC that the FBI will lead the investigation and would like to know contamination levels around the city to determine where it has safe (clean) access.

The mayor declares a local emergency and requests support from the state and federal governments.

The mayor and the governor hold a joint news conference and estimate that 50,000 people are affected by the evacuation. [*This number should be adjusted on the basis of the size of the jurisdiction.*]

The governor requests a presidential declaration of a federal disaster and orders the National Guard to mobilize.

Because of the exposure to radioactivity, all initial responders suffer from acute radiation exposure and many may die.

The 6 missing employees of [*incident site tenant company*] are still unaccounted for and are presumed to be dead; 10 employees are confirmed dead.

The president issues a disaster declaration. The Federal Response Plan and Federal Radiological Emergency Response Plan are activated.

FEMA and other federal agencies take active roles in the response.

FEMA activates the Emergency Response Team and deploys the advanced element of the Emergency Response Team and Federal Agency Support Team to the scene.

Some 2,500 people request medical treatment from area hospitals for radiation exposure.

Thousands of other people are reporting to hospitals claiming that they are sick or just wanting to be tested.

An initial assessment is conducted and elliptical contours are determined.

The fire at the incident site is extinguished.

Scene II: Chaos in the City

It is still [*day, date of the incident in the scenario*] in [*city, state, of the incident in the scenario state*]. The weather remains [*repeat previous forecast*]. The temperature is currently [*forecasted midday temperature, in degrees Fahrenheit, for the scenario*] with an expected high of [*forecasted high temperature, in degrees Fahrenheit, for the scenario*].

By 2:15 p.m. (1415 hours) the presence of a radioactive release is confirmed at the site. Readings indicate an exposure level of 60 rems/hour at the site. An immediate evacuation of the affected area is ordered. Mayor [*the name of the mayor*] says that [*he or she*] will talk with the governor soon and would like an update on evacuation, monitoring, and containment efforts as soon as possible to provide the governor with information.

On the basis of the information that it has received, the FBI believes that the device is a radioactivity dispersion device. The [*location of the closest FBI office*] office of the FBI notifies the city EOC that the FBI will take the lead in managing the crisis. It requests information about contamination levels around the city as soon as it is available to determine when it may access the site of the incident. The FBI wants to meet with representatives from the police department immediately to coordinate investigation efforts. It also requests that witnesses at or around the site be contacted and held for questioning by its investigators.

By 2:30 p.m. (1430 hours), the mayor declares a local emergency and asks the governor for assistance from the state and federal governments. Mayor [*full name of the mayor*] and Governor [*full name of governor*] subsequently hold a news conference. The governor indicates that [*he or she*] has declared a state of emergency and that an evacuation is in progress. City residents not evacuated are asked to remain indoors. Approximately 50,000 people are evacuated. [*This number should be adjusted on the basis of the size of the jurisdiction participating in this training activity.*]

The governor requests a presidential declaration of a federal disaster according to the Stafford Act. The governor orders the National Guard to mobilize to assist with the response effort.

Community health coordinators report that most initial emergency responders suffer from acute radiation exposure. The doctors anticipate that most, if not all, will die as a result of their exposure to high dosages of radiation. The six missing employees from the incident site remain unaccounted for and are presumed dead. Only 10 deaths are confirmed at this time.

The president issues a disaster declaration, promising to bring federal resources to respond to the emergency and to bring the responsible terrorists to justice. The Federal Response Plan and Federal Radiological Emergency Response Plan are activated. FEMA and other federal agencies are asked to provide assistance to the response and recovery processes. FEMA activates the Emergency Response Team and deploys the advanced elements of the Emergency Response Team and Federal Agency Support Team to the scene. Potential sites for the Disaster Field Office (DFO) are investigated.

Area hospitals report that more than 2,500 people have requested medical treatment because they believe they have been exposed to radiation. The few hospitals not under evacuation notices are overwhelmed with thousands of people claiming to suffer from radiation sickness or just wanting radiation exposure tests. Some of them do not have the resources to conduct the required tests or carry out treatment of any type, nor are they able to institute any kind of system to monitor people coming to the hospital.

Initial assessment survey reports indicate the following:

the elliptical contour for the 60-rem/hour dose extends 1 kilometer (km) in length and 500 meters in width from the site of the incident;

the elliptical contour for the 30-rem/hour dose is 2 km in length by 1 km in width;

the elliptical contour for the 15-rem/hour dose is 5 km in length and 2 km in width; and

the elliptical contour for the 10-rem/hour dose is 8 km in length and 3 km in width.

As a result of this information, the survey teams recommend that the evacuation area be increased. The areas of contamination now include:

[*Provide a bullet listing of the areas and major facilities and activities, e.g., hospitals and government buildings, contained within the contaminated area.*]

[*If possible, provide the participants with a map of the city with the contour lines marked on the map.*]

Thanks to heroic efforts of the fire department, the fire at the incident site is extinguished.

The rush of agencies descending on the scene is causing great confusion in command, control, and reporting. Confusion also exists in prioritizing response actions versus investigatory actions, leaving many responders upset. The area telephone system is overloaded, leading to concerns that the system may fail. Calls to the affected areas are not going through.

Questions, Scene II

1. Who is in charge of the incident site? How will your agency's actions be coordinated with the actions of other agencies? What conflicts could arise from the need to simultaneously conduct extensive criminal investigatory and response functions? What conflicts may be anticipated between the overlapping federal, state, and local jurisdictions?

Explore the federal definitions of crisis and consequence management. At the federal level, the FBI has authority over the incident site and is responsible for crisis management. FEMA has federal authority for consequence management, but must conform to the direction of the FBI to protect as much of the crime scene as possible while assisting local and state authorities with providing the needed rescue and relief to protect the population. It is anticipated that most jurisdictions will follow this delineation of responsibilities.

Determine who is in charge of the local response for both consequence and crisis management.

Determine the command or management structure to be used by the jurisdiction. The incident command system has been adapted by many jurisdictions as their command structure during response operations. Explore the specifics of the local system during this discussion. A review of the EOP should have provided details on the structure of the command structure.

Conflicts will likely be related to the jurisdiction's attempt to balance the protection of evidence and the protection of people. Overlapping conflicts can occur as state and federal responders arrive on scene and the transition to a unified, joint, or coordinated command or management structure begins.

The disposal of nuclear and radioactive materials is the responsibility of the U.S. Department of Energy. The U.S. Department of Energy should be involved in the control of contamination remaining at decontamination sites and will be responsible for its subsequent disposal.

2. What community health planning has been completed? Have privately owned hospitals, home-care agencies, long-term-care facilities, and clinics been incorporated into the EOP and included in the planning process? Has your community conducted joint exercises for this type or any type of mass-casualty situation?

The EOP review should indicate the preparedness of the community health program to address mass-casualty situations and the involvement of all local health care assets in the planning process.

Most jurisdictions should have been involved in joint mass-casualty exercises because these are an accreditation requirement for most health care organizations, especially hospitals.

Follow-up Questions:

What on-scene medical operations might be necessary?

This issue should be addressed in the community health plan as it exists. The priorities at the scene should be gross triage, transportation, and limited lifesaving efforts.

Will triage stations be established? Where will these be established?

The discussion of triage should focus on managing the flow of casualties through the community health system. The community health plan should address this issue.

What types of communications should be conducted between responders and the hospitals before the arrival of exposed victims? How will exposed patients be processed at point of collection and point of delivery?

Communications protocols for providing critical information should be provided within the communications section of the EOP.

Triage protocols at both collection and delivery points should also be part of the plan. Basic requirements dictate that triage be performed at both locations. This may be a good point to address the differences between standard emergency department triage and mass-casualty triage.

What specific assistance do you need from the state and federal governments? How will these resources be integrated into the response operations?

State and federal plans provide for mobilizing these types of resources in disaster situations. It is important for the group to realize that there may be a significant time delay before those resources are available.

What type of epidemiological surveillance program does your community have in place? How well defined are the linkages between the community health program and plan and your consequence management infrastructure?

Epidemiological surveillance is important in determining the number of individuals who were exposed to the radiological material. Community health planning should account for locating within the incident area personnel who may be asymptomatic at this point, especially in light of the potential long-term health effects.

The community should consider establishing a database to track the health of those members of the community, including responders, who may have been exposed to plutonium.

The EOP should define the linkage between the community health program and the emergency operations management structure, and a representative of the community health agency or emergency medical services should be on the management team.

3. What immediate public relations and media concerns must be anticipated? How will these concerns be addressed? Who will serve as your jurisdiction's spokesperson in this incident?

The Joint Information Center should be established after the arrival of state and federal assets and should serve as the source of pubic information after that point. The plan should identify who will serve as the local spokesperson before the establishment of the Joint Information Center.

Most EOPs assign the management of public affairs issues to the management team located in the EOC. Determine participants' familiarity with public affairs procedures. Anticipating that public panic and extreme fear are likely to exist, the group should discuss how to diffuse the issue without denigrating the seriousness of the situation. Determine if the participants understand the importance of a multimedia approach and the development of themes.

In the early stages of a response, public safety messages must be disseminated quickly.

Follow-up Question:

Does the communications system meet the multilingual needs of the area?

The EOP review should identify the multilingual needs of the community and procedures for meeting those needs.

4. What are the internal and external communications requirements for this response? Who is responsible for ensuring that the necessary systems are available? What problems may be anticipated?

The EOP should address internal and external communications requirements and assign responsibility for maintaining a viable system. Communications support equipment is normally located in or adjacent to the EOC.

Internal communications issues focus on the ability of jurisdictions to communicate with responders from different agencies (e.g., fire departments talking to police). Determine what system is in place to facilitate such coordination or if coordination must be accomplished face to face, through dispatchers, or through the EOC.

External communications issues should focus on the procedures for providing essential information to state and federal responders and managers who are en route to the incident site.

Solutions that rely on public hard telephone lines or cellular telephone systems should be discouraged in light of the numerous demands that will be made on those systems, unless the plan review revealed that a priority override system for emergency communications is in place with local telephone service providers.

Instructor's Background Information on the Incident, Scene III

With the downpour of rain, much of the radioactive particles are washed into the soil and down the [*appropriate name*] River, which flows from [*direction of river flow, e.g., south to north, if a river is in the area*]. [*If there is not a river in the area, describe the watershed and provide an indication of the potential areas that will be affected by the runoff.*] Farmers in [*provide names of locations in the area potentially affected by the runoff of radioactive particles*] use the irrigation water that has its source in this area.

Sanitation is a major issue at shelters and hospitals. The safety and health of patients who were in the hospitals for other reasons are compromised by the influx of patients and material contaminated with radioactive fallout.

Highlights of this scene include the following:

It starts getting dark and rainy.

The National Guard arrives and begins to take up positions throughout the city.

Hospitals request assistance with transporting overflow patients to other facilities.

Evacuated hospitals also request transportation and other logistical support.

Disposal of contaminated equipment and other material becomes a major issue.

Farmers downstream of the city are concerned about radiation fallout and its effect on their water supplies.

The public is provided with information on radiation exposure and fallout.

Reports indicate that approximately 3,800 people suffer radiation sickness or were exposed and require decontamination.

The DFO is situated, staffed, and in full operation.

The Joint Information Center is inundated with calls from the media about the response effort and the lack of information being provided to them.

Scene III: The Immediate Threat Wanes

It is 7:45 p.m. (1945 hours) on [*day, date of the incident in the scenario*] in [*city, state, of the incident in the scenario*]. The sun sets at [*appropriate time*]. Rain starts to fall. The temperature is currently [*forecasted temperature, in degrees Fahrenheit, at the end of the day*]. [*Since it is now evening, adjust the background description to the past tense if the sun has already set.*]

The rain and darkness complicate the response efforts. By 7:50 p.m. (1950 hours), members of the National Guard arrive and take up positions in and around downtown to assist the police with their duties and the decontamination and containment efforts. The American Red Cross offers assistance in transporting food, water, medications, and other resources to shelter locations and wherever else they are needed. Officials from the EPA contact the [*city or jurisdiction*] Public Works Department, [*city or jurisdiction*] Safety Department, and the [*state*] Department of Safety to coordinate efforts to monitor radiological contamination that may migrate into drinking water sources, surrounding lakes, rivers, and soil.

Several hospitals request assistance with transporting patients to other hospitals because of inadequate resources. They also request immediate assistance with monitoring incoming patients and decontamination procedures or they will be forced to turn additional patients away. Proper disposal of contaminated equipment and other material accumulating at the hospitals becomes a concern. The community health spokesperson [*or some other official, determined on the basis of an Office of Emergency Preparedness review*] holds a new conference at which he or she provides the public information regarding the effects of radiation under the current situation and encourages people to stay indoors. This conference is not coordinated with the Joint Information Center.

Agricultural, health, and safety officials from [*area, e.g., the state or surrounding counties*] and [*surrounding states*] are concerned that radiation fallout in the surrounding watershed, used for irrigation and other water supplies, will affect livestock and crops. Those calls persist as politicians from those areas pressure the EPA and the U.S. Department of Agriculture to certify the quality of the water from the region.

By 10:30 p.m. (2230 hours), updated reports of casualties filter in from area hospitals, shelters, and residences. It is reported that approximately 3,800 people either suffer radiation sickness or were exposed to radiation and still require decontamination and advanced medical treatment.

U.S. Department of Defense, U.S. Department of Energy, and EPA officials express concern about the possibility of a large number of people leaving the area before being monitored for contamination. There is also concern that many contaminated vehicles traveled to other jurisdictions.

By 4 a.m. (0400 hours), the DFO is in full operation. The media inundates the Joint Information Center with calls questioning the adequacy of the response effort and the lack of information provided to them and the public by state and local authorities.

The FBI requests protective equipment to access the site of the explosion to look for clues and extract the remains of the radioactivity dispersion device.

Questions, Scene III

1. How will you conduct extended response operations? Are local personnel and equipment resources adequate for the extended operations that will be required?

The EOP should account for around-the-clock operations. Many jurisdictions plan to send a portion of the EOC staff home after the initial incident assessment reveals the need for extended operations. Determine who will be responsible for each function on multiple shifts.

Each agency will likely be overwhelmed. The real questions are how much state, federal, National Guard, and mutual-aid support is needed.

2. What are your procedures for integrating state and federal resources into your management organization?

The EOP should outline the procedures for state and federal integration.

State and federal assistance is supplementary to the local response; and as the DFO is established the federal coordinating officer and state coordinating officer will coordinate the activities of the state and local governments, the American Red Cross, the Salvation Army, and other disaster relief organizations.

Follow-up Questions:

How will your agency coordinate its action with other agencies (federal, state, and local) and public interest groups?

The federal coordination officer is the primary federal coordinating authority for consequence management; the FBI handles crisis management.

With the arrival of state and federal assistance and the formation of a Joint Information Center, how will media inquiries be handled? Who in your jurisdiction is responsible for authoring media releases?

Media releases must be coordinated with the FBI, FEMA, and state and local authorities once the Joint Information Center has been established.

The EOP should provide a detailed communications and public relations plan.

3. What continuing assessments should be enacted when the cleanup phase is complete? Who will make these determinations?

Long-range health issues are of great concern.

Hazmat sites, especially decontamination stations, should be examined periodically until it is determined that there is no longer an environmental hazard.

The EOP should provide an overview of how continuing assessments and long-term monitoring are accomplished; allow the participants in the group to discuss their areas of concern and propose priorities.

4. What are the environmental concerns related to this incident?

There are numerous concerns related to plutonium, for example, it is a heavy metal and is toxic in its own right beyond the long-term effects on humans, animals, and other forms of life. The local responders might also identify some issues particular to their area.

Materials used during the response will continue to present hazards until they are neutralized.

Follow-up Questions:

What steps will be taken by your agency to ensure adequate sanitation measures throughout the affected area?

The local hazmat plan should identify sanitation procedures related to radiological operations.

What local requirements exist for reentry to an evacuated area due to a hazmat incident?

The hazmat annex to the EOP should outline reentry procedures.

After the release of radioactive materials, the local emergency management team should consider the need for safe certification, that is, having a third-party laboratory verify that the area is free from contamination.

5. Within your jurisdiction, what psychological traumas may be anticipated? How will your agency deal with these traumas?

Many agencies have teams already designated to assist in such cases. In most instances, the teams will not have the capacity to handle the expected number of cases in an incident of this magnitude.

Discuss the availability of crisis counseling. Also, refer participants to Section 416 of the Stafford Act.

Follow-up Questions:

How will your agency participate in notification of the deaths of civilians and your colleagues? Are personnel in your agency adequately trained in the process of death notification?

Death notification is always a difficult issue. The EOP should provide guidance to managers. However, at a minimum someone in the supervisory chain should be involved with the actual notification.